# The Keto Autoimmune Protocol Healing Book for Women

Sometimes struggles are exactly what our life needs. After you walk through the valley, you really appreciate the mountain top– A.L. Childers

"Fall in love with oneself, be aware and in control of what your nourishing your body and learn thyself" – A.L. Childers

"It would depend on the taste of the observer which he now wishes to regard as real"- Erwin Schrödinger 1926

"Toxins from food and the environment can make you fat. Toxins may come in the form of medication, bacteria, industrial chemicals, and heavy metals. These pollutants can damage or block the signals that control your appetite. You can detoxify your body with the right balance of protein, fats, fiber, vitamins, minerals, and phytonutrients found in plant foods."

– Dr. Mark Hyman

My darling, you cannot talk butterfly language with caterpillar people

Begin your day with by thanking God for all he has done for you. Your bed you sleep in, your clean sheets, your water, anything that you have whether it is big or small. Why would God give you more if you're ungrateful for what he has given you already? Stop blocking your blessings. Slowly inhale, verbally speak out loud and thank God for all he has given you and what he will give you. Ask, Believe and receive.

-A.L. Childers

Dedication:

This book has been dedicated to my Beautiful niece Brittany who never ceases to amaze me. She's a proud active member in our military, wonderful mother of a brilliant, creative and full of personality daughter named Antonia.

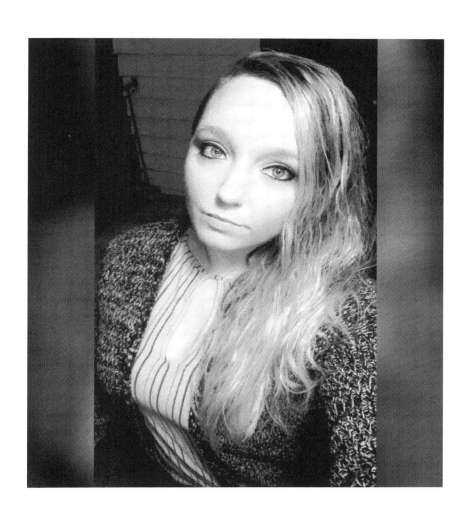

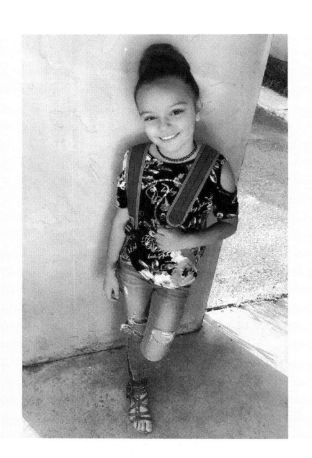

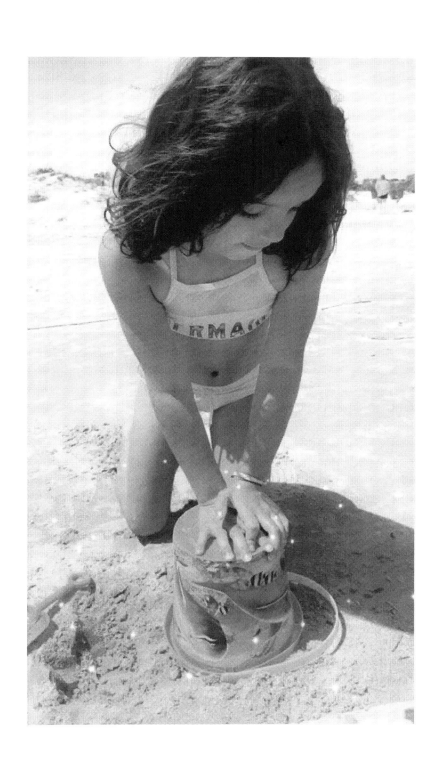

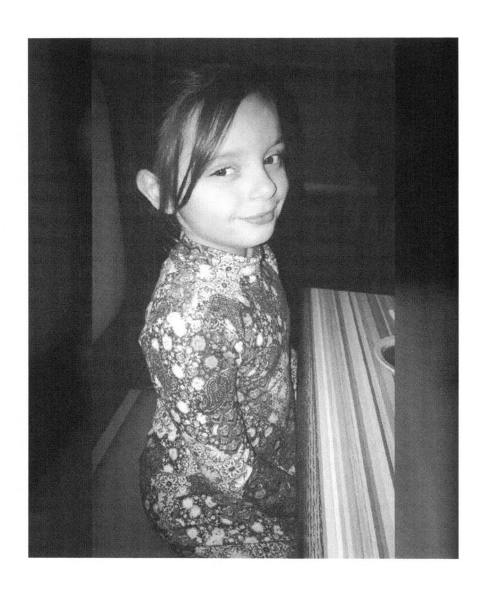

## Hey You, Beautiful:

I feel more fueled than ever in my mission to help empower others to take control of their health. Conditions will never be perfect to begin your health journey; there will always be reasons to put things off for another day. Don't let perfection or fear keep you from beginning your journey and don't let obstacles stop you along the way. You have the power to change. And today is the day to begin. Let's not forget that we are all different. Each one of us are unique and we are biochemically individually wired and what works for one person may not work for another. We are extremely complex and each person should be valued independently. My reason for having a leaky gut, inflammation and an autoimmune disorder might not be your reason. Each day we encounter is different for each of us. Every Cell in your body responds to the foods you eat, the products you put on your body to the house hold chemicals that you purchase for your home. All of these things have a direct impact on your hormones and in return your hormones have a direct impact on every major system in your body. Life isn't a 1 size fits all solution. I want to try to help you understand the many debilitating aspects of having these medical conditions. This book is packed full of wonderful information and is meant to be an eye opener for everyone who wants to make a difference in their lives. I hope that you will allow this book to be just one of your resources that is empowering you to try to help make sense of it all.

"Every time you
Eat or drink,
You are either
Feeding
disease or fighting it"

A note of caution:

I strongly support self-care, personal health empowerment and improving your understanding of thyroid health. However, this cannot substitute by a trained medical professional in cases of long standing and undiagnosed symptoms. This book is thus not meant as a substitute for professional medical judgement, though it can serve as a helpful adjunct to it. All content within this book is commentary or opinion and is protected under Free Speech laws in all the civilized world. The information herein is provided for educational and entertainment purposes only

When in doubt about your thyroid seek your doctor or your medical professional to exclude serious medical conditions. It is not intended as a substitute for professional advice of any kind. Audrey Childers assumes no responsibility for the use or misuse of this material.

Therefore no warranty of any kind, whether expressed or implied, is given in relation to this information. This is a comprehensive limitation of liability that applies to all damages of any kind, including (without limitation) compensatory; direct, indirect or consequential damages; loss of data, income or profit; loss of or damage to property and claims of third parties.

Be safe, be sane and be healthy.

Get a complete exam from a reliable health practitioner. Do what you can do within the boundaries of good common sense.

In a word, be kind to yourself and your body.

A.L. Childers

Disclaimer:

The information and recipes contained in this book are based upon the research and the personal experiences of the author. This is my opinion, since many other authorities may say something different--not necessarily about the potential action of eating KETO AIP, but the whole picture of what to eat and how to change your life for the better. It's for entertainment purposes only. It is not meant to replace any advice from a health care professional. This book is meant to compliment. The reader is encouraged to use good judgement when apply the information contained and to seek advice from a qualified professional if, and as, needed. Every attempt has been made to provide accurate, up to date and reliable information. No warranties of any kind are expressed or implied. Readers acknowledge that the author is not engaging in the rendering of legal, financial, medical or professional advice. This way of eating isn't for everyone. Normally your body burns carbohydrates for fuel. When you drastically cut carbs, the body goes into a metabolic state called ketosis, and it begins to burn its own fat for fuel. Please check with your doctor to make sure you can eat a lower carb, higher protein diet. Low-carb diets may help prevent or improve serious health conditions, such as metabolic syndrome, diabetes,

# *From the Author:*

Educating and learning how your body works is one of the most important tools that you can learn. Sure, some of the information contained in this book isn't anything really new that you haven't heard before and one simply could of did their own research on any website about women and health to find many of the topics covered throughout this book.

What you won't find researched on any website is how insightful this book is based from my own experiences.

Look, I don't have good genes. The people in my southern family have diabetes, heart disease and cancer has been rampant. I've had to fight for good health. Sometimes, I felt as if I had fallen down an abandoned water well and been trapped for days trying to climb my way out but with each attempt, even when I have almost climbed my way to the top; Only to slip again as I fall swiftly and violently all the way back down in the cold, shallow, murky water below. I am just left with the thoughts of how I am going to die here and no one will ever know. This book is more than anything you can simply read on a website. Do you feel as if you're trapped too? Everything you have done up until this point, is just not working. All the years of struggling and research has led me to this point. The journey of my health and the history of my family's health has led me to this point. I want to break that curse that has been passed down in my family's genes. I don't have a registered dietitian nutritionist label nor a PHD behind my name but I can share with you what has happened in my life and what has worked for me. My journey, my walk and my candid openness. Expertise doesn't always come with a degree. We are in the midst of a huge battle, my friends. The things they allow to be placed in our food are inhumane and is quite frankly killing us.

Humans have evolved to become one of the smartest species on the planet but yet we have become dumbfounded on how to correctly nourish our bodies or have we just become so busy, well, I hate to say this but have we become "to lazy" and just got in the cycle of grabbing what is convenient? We certainly haven't *forgotten* how to eat food but somewhere along the way we became confused to what is real food or do we even care? We are consuming food like products and truthfully we are enjoying every single mouthful although it is slowly poisoning our bodies and damaging our DNA. Food is not just calories, it is information. This information talks to your DNA and tells it what to do. One of the most powerful tools to change your health is your fork. If you keep feeding your DNA the wrong information it's not going to know how to process it. If it can't dispose of it, it will begin to start storing it in random places and your body will eventually begin to break down.

There are a lot of misguided and confusing information out there regarding nutrition we seem to be eager to try the next health fad in hopes of dropping pounds, improving our health and healing what ails us. A big misconception is that fat makes you fat. There is good fat and there is bad fat. Not all fats are created equal. Our bodies need the "good" dietary fat. Many people are baffled by which fats should we be eating because the U.S. Dietary Guidelines (and nutrition labels) are misleading and according to a research done by the University of Maryland Medical Center, "Most Americans are getting 20x's the amount of omega-6s than we really need". This is the bad type of fat. This is the type of saturated fat that you eat that will make you fat like pizza, burgers, processed foods, processed snacks and sweets. We should be consuming more of the Omega 3 fat's which are minimally-processed and full of heart-healthy, polyunsaturated omega-3 fatty acids (ALA, DHA, and EPA), monounsaturated fats

(OEA), and the trans-fat conjugated linoleic acid (CLA), as well as some medium-chain saturated fats like stearic acid and lauric acid. Examples of these goods fats are Wild Salmon, Olive Oil, Avocado, Coconut and Grass-Fed Beef.

For some reason we have been conditioned and programmed to believe that low-fat and fat-free products are healthier. These foods that are low-fat or fat-free are refined, overly processed foods, loaded with fake ingredient's that were created in a lab and full of sugar.

The typical American Standard diet lacks nutrients that are absolutely essential for good health. Most of us know that we are all unique in every aspect of our lives. Your body requires many different vitamins and minerals that are crucial for both remaining healthy and preventing disease. No matter what lifestyle change you decide to attempt you will find that every single diet will have deficiencies aka (Malnutrition). It seems with this day in age we shouldn't have an issue with our plates not being a complete balanced meal with real based foods. A balanced diet won't mean the same to everyone. We are all unique in every aspect of our lives. We all do have a similar cellular structure that ensures growth, body maintenance and specific functions but many disorders have a direct or indirect connection caused by the lack of proper nutrition. People's health disorders can be caused by a person's genetic make-up, lifestyle behavior's (e.g. smoking, drinking, and drugs), and exposure to toxic substances (e.g. asbestos, household chemicals, pesticides) or other reasons not mentioned. This is why I say," We are all unique in every aspect of our lives." As of 2012, about half of all adults—117 million people— had one or more chronic health conditions. One in four adults had two or more chronic health conditions. One health problem or illness can lead to another. It's like a domino effect. There is a distinct difference between treating the symptoms and curing the condition. Sometimes the reason for your illness is as plain as the nose on your face. For example; Sally can link her COPD (Chronic Obstructive Pulmonary Disease) and heart disease to 25 years of smoking. Thomas can link his stomach cancer to the radiation he was exposed to from his work history. Lucy's irregular heart beat could have been caused by her excess alcohol habit. Then there are times when you have no idea why you are sick and you can't pin point the reason. Micronutrients aren't produced naturally in the body, therefore we have to get them from our diets. You have a unique physiology that must be supported properly with an individualized approach that includes proper nutrition and supplementation. This book can help you begin to understand what an AIP Keto protocol is and start guiding you in the redevelopment and healing of your body. It also will begin to fix your gut, strengthen your immunity and fight inflammation with an autoimmune approach. Along with helping to reset those adrenals, boosting that energy and doing a little ass kicking to those hormones that have decided to act like a wild college student and pull an all-nighter the day before final exams.

Your health doesn't have to be a difficult situation but a positive realization that things need to change. This journey that you are on will have many parts to it and I hope you will embrace not only the physical but also the spiritual awakening.

Remember, awareness has magic and health is truly your wealth.

Thehypothyroidismchick.com

A.L. Childers is available for speaking engagements.

To inquire, please send an email to Audreychilders@hotmail.com

I created this personal contract. I hope you will print it and use it to your best ability. Your Personal Contract

I..........................................................................................
......

Declare that I will master my life in every aspect of it. I will no longer settle for less than I deserve. I have the courage, will power and wisdom to know that it's my time to make a difference in my life. I will put my best foot forward in all areas of my life. I will wake up grateful, put the right foods in my body for nourishment and uplift others.

I am the only person responsible for my life and I believe with every fiber of my being that that I can make a difference.

I am enough. I will be true to myself and follow my heart. My personal development is in my own hands AND I will stop fighting against myself. I will stop listening to self-doubt. My past experiences will not affect my current mindset. God will support me in with joyful abundance in all areas of my life. This book is only the beginning of my wonderful journey to happiness, joy, peace and prosperity. I am willing to go beyond my past and I am the only person who chooses my path and I don't need anyone's approval. I release all limitations from my past.

I will seek the highest truth and the most healing ways to live my life. Health and Happiness is abundantly mine.

Love,

Signed by ………………

# The Connection between Food and Autoimmune disorders

Our body's immune response is a marvelous defense system. It protects against foreign invaders, injury, and infection through a complex communication system between your body's cells and the chemical signals they produce. If you have a healthy immune system, this communication is clear and specific; the body can tell the difference between an itself and a foreigner invader.

An autoimmune disease is any condition where a person's immune system has an abnormal immune response and mistakenly attacks itself along with damaging its own bodily tissues. This leaves the immune response is flawed, and the communication system breaks down where it can't distinguish the body's tissues from foreign cells.

Close to 24 million (7%) people in the United States are affected by an autoimmune disease and scientists have identified more than 80 clinically distinct autoimmune diseases.

Autoimmunity is the No. 2 cause of chronic illness, according to the American Autoimmune Related Diseases Association (AARDA), a nonprofit health agency dedicated to increasing awareness of autoimmune diseases. Autoimmune diseases can affect nearly every part of the body.

There was a study done by The Multiple Autoimmune Disease Genetics Consortium (MADGC) in 1999. In this study, they describe a unique collection of 65 families comprising 300-400 individuals.  To qualify, a family must have at least two of the eight autoimmune diseases chosen for the study. These core diseases include rheumatoid arthritis (RA), systemic lupus erythematosus (SLE), type 1 diabetes (T1D), multiple sclerosis (MS), autoimmune thyroid disease (Hashimoto thyroiditis or Graves' disease), juvenile RA, inflammatory bowel disease

(Crohn disease or ulcerative colitis), psoriasis, and primary Sjögren syndrome. The main objective was to see if they could identify genes that several autoimmune diseases have in common.

The researchers followed these families around for 5 years and taking detailed histories through mailings and office visits, researchers hope to get some idea of pertinent environmental factors, and which ones appear to be most relevant to which genetic profiles. Factors likely to be scrutinized include infectious and noninfectious agents, drugs, vaccines, food, dietary supplements, organic solvents, ultraviolet light, stress and stressful life events, and occupational exposures. They found there was a common between autoimmunity and inflammation that couldn't be ignored. Inflammation helped to set the stage per say for everything else to fall into place. You certainly dont have to study tens and tens of thousands of people to see an association with an environmental factor.

So, what is the connection between Food and Autoimmunity. There is this big lie that we have all got stuck in and we are not looking at the most obvious solution.

All of this abuse on our bodies is disrupting our body's normal rhythms from being able to function properly. There is scientific evidence available that support the effectiveness of the AIP diet in the management and treatment of autoimmune diseases.

Food is thy medicine and the old saying is true; We are what we eat?

Food can be thy medicine or food can be thy death. The truth is the foods that we are consuming are creating an epidemic of illness in America. We are actually nutrient starved and very malnourished. American's are suffering from over consumption of refined oils, refined grains and these processed foods like food products. The typical American Standard diet lacks nutrients that are absolutely essential for overall good health.

If we are what we eat? Just because you consumed food today doesn't mean what you consumed put any needed nutrition in your body, gave your body the needed fuel to perform correctly, and reduce your risk of chronic diseases.

Your gut is your portal to health. It houses 80 percent of your immune system, and without your gut being healthy it is practically impossible to have a healthy immune system. A properly working digestive system (your gut) is vital to your health.

Did you know that your gut is the largest component of your immune system? Around 1,000 different species of bugs live in your gut. Your gut has been linked to contributing to weight loss and for overall improvement of numerous symptoms, including depression, anxiety, brain fog, skin problems, hormonal issues, immune weaknesses, digestive problems, fatigue and of course the elephant in the room; Autoimmune disorders.

Inflammation is one of the common traits of an autoimmune disease. You must eliminate the foods that may be causing inflammation in the gut.

Think about what you're putting in your body. Either you're fighting disease or feeding disease. You must get a concept of nutrient density. Gluten, dairy and soy products create inflammation in the digestive tract. If you have inflammation in the digestive system undigested proteins leak into the blood stream creating a heightened immune reaction that often makes issues worse and can lead to a leaky gut which causes other problems.

When undigested proteins leak into the blood stream creating a heightened immune reaction.

# Finding Your Food Code

In the last fifty years what has changed in our society? We have the same predisposition genetics as our grandparents. We are unique and come in all different shapes, sizes, race, religions and greed.

We can't blame is all on genetics being unhealthy solely on the DNA that was passed down to us. Everyone's genetic makeup is different. It's like your fingerprints.

Let me say this a little bit louder so the people in the back row can hear...

YOUR GENES ARE NOT YOUR DESTINY!

Yes, every cell in our body responds to how you live, eat, sleep, move, think, feel, and breathe determines whether you turn those genetic switches on or off. It's called epigenetics.

It's up to you. Decide. It's up to us to break generation curses.

When you hear someone say, "it runs in the family". You reply, "this is where it runs out".

Our metabolisms certainly dictate how we use energy and our genetics can dictate how we are shaped along with other traits. One thing we have learned is each of us are unique and have our very own biochemistry that sets us apart from everyone else. Although we might share the same common traits and perhaps the same overlapping metabolic tendencies. We can't continue to say that one-size-fits-all when it comes to our very own unique body chemistry. There are over 7 billion people on this planet and we come in all different shapes, colors and sizes. With this being said wouldn't you think the one-size-fits-all- approach to losing weight wouldn't work since we are we are all unique. Also, with this all being said wouldn't you think that we all have our very own personal food code too?

Although some of us were born with the predisposition genetics as our parents that gives us our hair color, eye color, height and if we are pear shaped, apple shaped, straight or hourglass this doesn't mean we can't win the battle when it comes to our hormones. Our hormones have a direct impact on every major system in our body.
Remember our bodies love balance.
Everything has a domino effect so we have to try to figure-out that balance in what our individual body needs are. Whether it be the more fiber , fixing our gut, helping our skin get more moisture, speeding up our metabolism so we can get out of that fat storage mode and into the fat burning mode.

Finding your food code won't be as easy as it sounds. Quite frankly you will have to put some elbow grease into this but it's not unattainable. How we live from day to day is completely different on every spectrum across the board. One thing I do know for-sure is that every single day no matter who we are or where we live our bodies are bombarded with a toxic burden of chemicals, we are not feeding our bodies the proper nutrients, we are nutritional deficient, and some of us have little to no activity & these are some of the reasons why our bodies are becoming stagnant and increasingly polluted. It would be silly to take Motrin for a rock stuck in your shoe when all you had to do was pluck it out. So why not on this journey go ahead, do some research and start addressing the issues at hand.

We are creating a perfect storm within our bodies. The less nutrients we consume, more toxins we add, create this world win of health issues. It's sad that our western diet is made up of hormone filled meats, vegetable oils, white flour and sugar. Who would have thought that something so simple as eating has become so complicated? Food does matter.

It talks to your DNA.

Food can change your DNA!

The foods you eat have a major impact your life — It affects your gut health and along with increasing or decreasing the inflammation in your body. Unfortunately, our western world diet are full of foods that have a bad impact on both your gut and your inflammation.  If it was made in a lab, avoid it. Do a little research and you will find that our western diet that is made up of processed, fake foods, chemicals, sugar and corn oils are all highly flaming the fan of your inflammation.

We have a shortage of nutrients in our food system. The most common foods that you load up your grocery cart with are loaded with bad carbs, fillers, preservatives, additives, flavorings, and chemicals. Your body doesn't have any idea what do to with all this fake food. We are creating a weaker human race, inflammation and pain along with the possibility of welcoming other diseases and disorders. Your diet and lifestyle choices is what has caused any health issues that you may have unless you were born with a health issue then you can look at your parents diet , surroundings and lifestyle choices. It can go back generations. The only way to get back our health and vitality is to look at the root of it all.

# You can change and control your life.

Think about what you're putting in your body. Either you're fighting disease or feeding disease. You must get a concept of nutrient density.  Gluten, dairy and soy products create inflammation in the digestive tract. In ancient times grains were prepared by soaking, sprouting and fermenting but that tradition in making them been long forgotten with our fast-paced culture.

*Healthy Cells Grow from the Inside Out*

# Processed Carbs
# and
# the Body

Not all carbs are created equal. Processed carbs is nothing more than empty calories. They have been stripped away of mostly all of the beneficial nutrients and natural fibers that your body needs for nourishment along with spiking your blood sugar quickly and stimulating insulin response. When you begin to start reading labels you will notices thinks like the word, "enriched" this was created to fool you into thinking that the product is okay to eat. What the manufacturers has actually done was chemically added certain nutrients back in to processed carbs with synthetic vitamins that can't even compare to the naturally-occurring beneficial nutrients and natural fibers in whole foods.

In a study published in the "American Journal of Clinical Nutrition" in February 2006, researchers analyzed the negative effects of processed carbs on 932 health men and women. Participants who ate Low-glycemic carbs showed a radical control of their blood sugar spikes, better cholesterol levels and no increase in inflammation.

Inflammation can become your enemy when it's been associated with leptin resistance, which is thought to be a major factor for obesity.  Also when you have chronic inflammation in your body your immune system goes into a protection mode because it doesn't recognize these fake foods and it feels it's under attack.

Chronic inflammation has been linked to major disease like cancer, heart disease, diabetes, arthritis, depression, and Alzheimer's.

This constant cycle can also set you up for metabolic syndrome and in-return begin to store harmful belly fat around your midsection giving you a lovely muffin top.

Your body adapts to what your feeding it, the nutrients that are supplied are being processed differently and are sent to where its need. Just like a car, each item has its own function and you can run a car efficiently without every part working as it should. The proteins, fats, and carbs are all converted into fuel using many different metabolic processes. Our bodies were not designed to eat foods like refined sugar, high fructose corn syrup, cereal, bread, potatoes and pasteurized milk products.

You see when your feed your body carbohydrates it will break it down and convert most of it into the sugar glucose. Glucose is then absorbed into the bloodstream, and with the help of a hormone called insulin it travels into the cells of the body where it can be used for energy. If there is any leftover glucose and more than the liver can hold it will be won't be wasted.

Your body will turn it into fat for overall storage for later use. You see if you don't have an overload of carbohydrates your body can and will run mainly on fats. We've been spoon fed by mainstream medical organizations to believe that glucose is the preferred fuel of our metabolism but actually it is fat for fuel that is the key to ideal health. Nutritional Ketosis is actually a proven powerful method to burn fat for fuel instead of sugar for fuel.  When you burn fat for fuel you increase your energy, improve your mental clarity and sharpness, keeps your blood sugar stabilized, begin to balance your hormones, decrease inflammation, Increases levels of HDL Cholesterol (the good cholesterol), lowers your blood pressure, fights against Metabolic Syndrome and helps to clear your skin. One hour after consuming refined carbs your Blood sugar levels drop and signals the brain that its needs to be stimulated again by more refined carbs.

There are two main forms of carbohydrates:

Simple carbohydrates which are foods such as fructose, glucose, and lactose. These carbs are easily and quickly utilized for energy by the body because of their simple chemical structure, often leading to a faster rise in blood sugar and insulin secretion from the pancreas – which can have negative health effects.

Complex carbohydrates which are foods contain fiber, vitamins and minerals, and they take longer to digest

We've been lied to again by American Academy of Nutrition and Dietetics, the American Diabetes Association, and other mainstream medical organizations. Eating complex carbs should not spike your blood sugar and it also should be healthy for us to consume. Normal blood sugar and insulin levels are vital to keeping our bodies healthy.

You don't get fat from eating good fats. In Dr. Richard Johnson, latest book, The Fat Switch, has proven by in his research that fructose activates a key enzyme, fructokinase, which in turn activates another enzyme that causes cells to accumulate fat. Another fabrication by the mainstream medical organizations that has been proven wrong about diet and obesity.

In 1931, German physician Dr. Otto Warburg discovered that cancer cells have a fundamentally different energy metabolism compared to healthy cells – a discovery that won him the Nobel Prize for Physiology or Medicine.

Warburg discovered cancer cells are primarily fueled by the burning of sugar anaerobically, and that most cancer cells do not have the metabolic flexibility to survive without sugar. A New York Times article notes:

The Warburg effect is estimated to occur in up to 80 percent of cancers. [A] Positron emission tomography (PET) scan, which has emerged as an important tool in the staging and diagnosis of cancer works simply by revealing the places in the body where cells are consuming extra glucose.

In many cases, the more glucose a tumor consumes, the worse a patient's prognosis."

Your body needs good carbs not bad processed carbs like grains, sugars and fake foods. Typical daily intake of good carbs can vary between 20 to 100 grams a day, and it all depends on if you are fat adapted to burn ketones (fat for fuel) and the amount of exercise you do. We are all individuals and each one of us are unique with our own metabolic and nutrition efficiency needs. We must begin to listen, become accountable and understand where our body are struggling to begin weight-loss and becoming healthier. There is no secret magical pill. It does take discipline, commitment and action. You cannot, no matter how hard you try do growth work for another person. This is your choice to decide to better your life and become healthy. Eating well isn't boring nor bland. Once you learn how to eat to nourish your body you are going to feel so much better.

# Sugar: The Hidden Epidemic

I grew up watching my single mother struggle to keep a roof over our heads and food on the table. Back in the early 80's, as she worked two jobs, she would give me $5 each day from her tips to go to the grocery store and purchase dinner for my sister who is 5 years younger than me. The Piggly Wiggly was just around the corner from our one-bedroom garage apt. I learned the value of money at an early age and the value of what to buy to keep us full until the next day when we would eat our free lunch at school. My mouth watered as I passed the junk food isle. Anything with sugar in it was a treat that I rarely had the chance to consume. Fast Forward twenty years later, without realizing it, until recently, I had become a food addict. Food felt good to me and made me forget about all those years listening to the sounds of my rumbling stomach. The daily struggle to eat as a child had developed a hidden childhood trauma inside of me. Once a person realizes they have a destructive-addictive behavior they can either do 1 of 2 things. Take control back or allow it to control you.

This is just my story but as you're reading this perhaps you can think back to a time in your past where you may just realize exactly where your addiction might have started.

The king of artificial sweeteners was allowed to the market in 1981 when the U.S. Commissioner of Food and Drugs, Arthur Hull Hayes, overruled FDA panel suggestions, as well as consumer concerns. Aspartame is a neurotoxin that interacts with natural organisms, as well as synthetic medications, producing a wide range of proven disorders and syndromes. So who installed this commissioner that would rule against scientists and the public? Donald Rumsfeld, CEO of G.D. Searle; the maker of Aspartame. Rumsfeld was on Reagan's transition team, and the day after Reagan took office he appointed the new FDA

Commissioner in order to "call in his markers" with one of the most egregious cases of profit-over-safety ever recorded.

Aspartame is now nearly ubiquitous, moving beyond sugarless products and into general foods, beverages, pharmaceuticals, and even products for children. It recently has been renamed to the more pleasant sounding Amino Sweet.

According to a Parent company survey with over 1500 participants one of the greatest fears as a parent is for their child to become addicted to drugs and alcohol but without even realizing it, many parents are raising addicts. Sugar addicts. Addiction can manifest in many forms therefore writing about sugar addiction has had its many challenges.

Sugar has no nutritional value and is nothing but empty calories and is hidden in everything that we eat that is processed or pre-packaged by mankind. Sugar is addictive like most modern day drugs and it activates the same brain system as drugs such as nicotine and cocaine. It is responsible for a large number of health conditions that plague humans in the 21st century.

Refined sugar doesn't contain any nutritional value. You won't find any fiber, vitamins, minerals, antioxidants, water, fats or proteins but what you will find is inflammation, malnutrition, bad carbohydrates, metabolic syndrome, blood sugar spikes, leptin resistance AND obesity.

Did you know? According to the American Heart Association (AHA), the maximum amount of sugar you should eat in a day is as follows:


Men: 150 calories per day (37.9 grams or 9 teaspoons)

Women: 100 calories per day (25 grams or 6 teaspoons)

Children 2-18 years old: 100 calories (25 grams or 6 teaspoons)

According to the National Cancer Institute and National Health and Nutrition Examination Survey, children as young as 1 to 3 years already exceed the daily recommendations and typically consume around 12 teaspoons of added sugar a day. By the time a child is 4 to 8 years old, his sugar intake soars to an average of 21 teaspoons a day.

The National Cancer Institute also found that 14- to 18-year-old children consume the most added sugar on a daily basis, averaging about 34.3 teaspoons. In general, the average American consumes about 355 calories of added sugar a day, or the equivalent of 22.2 teaspoons. That is about triple the recommended amount!

Look at the label of a standard can of soda.

| Serving Size 1 can (12 fl oz) | |
| Serving Per Container 1 | |

**Amount Per Serving**

**Calories** 140

| | % Daily Values* |
|---|---|
| **Total Fat** 0g | 0% |
| Saturated Fat 0g | 0% |
| Trans Fat 0g | |
| **Cholesterol** 0mg | 0% |
| **Sodium** 45mg | 2% |
| **Total Carbohydrate** 39g | 13% |
| Dietary Fiber 0g | 0% |
| Sugars 39g | |
| **Protein** 0g | 0% |

There are 39grams of sugar in this one can of soda. So how much exactly is a gram of sugar? One teaspoon of granulated sugar equals 4 grams of sugar. To put it another way, 16 grams of sugar in a product is equal to about 4 teaspoons of granulated sugar.

This one can of soda 35g of sugar amounts to about 7 teaspoons of sugar.

Here's how to calculate from calories to grams to teaspoons. Use the "divide by 4" rule of simple sugar math. Take the calories and divide by 4 to get the grams of added sugar. For example, 200 calories, this is 50 grams.

DelMonte diced pears or mandarin oranges in light syrup: 1 small serving cup = 17 grams' sugar, 70 calories (that's 5 teaspoons of sugar)

Quaker Instant Oatmeal, Strawberries & Cream or Peaches & Cream: 1 envelope = 12 grams' sugar, 130 calories (That's 2.75 teaspoons of sugar)

Prego Fresh Mushroom Italian Sauce: 1/2 cup = 11 grams' sugar, 90 calories (that's 2.75 teaspoons of sugar)

Snapple Iced Peach Tea:  16 ounces = 39 grams' sugar, 200 calories (that's 9.75 teaspoons of sugar)

Starbucks Carmel Frappuccino:  64 grams (that's 16 teaspoons of sugar)

# THE 56 NAMES OF
# SUGAR

Buttered syrup
Cane sugar
Dextrose
Caramel
Brown sugar
Corn syrup
Cane juice
Corn syrup solids
Beet sugar
Confectioners' sugar
Dehydrated cane juice
Galactose
Agave nectar
Demerara sugar
Fruit juice concentrate
Maltodextrin
Diastatic malt
Diatase
Maltose
Fructose
Malt sugar
Mannitol
Florida crystals
Molasses
Sucrose
Sorghum syrup
Sorbitol
Yellow sugar
Carob syrup
Treacle
Lactose
Panocha
Raw sugar
Rice syrup
Castor sugar
HFCS (High Frustose Corn Syrup)
Golden sugar
Muscovado
Barbados sugar
Glucose solids
Barley malt
Grape sugar
Maple syrup
Honey
Golden syrup
Refiner's Syrup
Sugar (granulated)
Turbinado sugar
Glucose
Date sugar
Fruit juice
Icing sugar
Dextran
Ethyl maltol

Circulation: Journal of the American Heart Association, a published article in August 2009 connected the increased sugar consumption with a variety of health problems like inflammation, including obesity and high blood pressure.

A new study published in the Journal of Clinical Investigation states that an excess of sugar on our liver is making our body's insulin resistance. And is the beginning stages of nonalcoholic fatty liver disease.

The excess of sugar fools our metabolism into turning off our body's appetite-control system.  When this happens the body doesn't stimulate insulin, which in turn fails to suppress ghrelin, or "the hunger hormone," which then fails to stimulate leptin or "the satiety hormone." This is what sets us up for insulin resistance, metabolic dysfunction, weight gain, abdominal obesity, decreased HDL and increased LDL, elevated blood sugar, elevated triglycerides, high blood pressure and more uric acid which place us in the risk factor for heart and kidney disease. All these things from the over consumption of sugar that is in processed foods.

Eating too much sugar has many negative effects on the body, such as putting you at risk for: Obesity, Insulin resistance, Type 2 diabetes, Fatty liver disease, and Certain types of cancer.

Dr. Robert Lustig, a professor of Clinical Pediatrics in the Division of Endocrinology in the University of California and a pioneer in decoding sugar metabolism, says that your body can safely metabolize at least six teaspoons of added sugar per day. Only 6 teaspoons but the average American is eating three times that amount.

I hope you can clearly see and have no misconceptions on why childhood obesity has become an epidemic in America. The World Health Organization estimate that there are 43 million overweight children who are under the age of 5. By 2020, more than 60 percent of diseases worldwide will be directly associated with obesity. According to research published in the Journal of Family Medicine and Primary Care, "childhood obesity can greatly affect a child's mental and physical health, along with their social, emotional and self-esteem well-being. The over-consumption of sugar also creates a viscous cycle of intense cravings and wreaks havoc on our brain.

The pharmaceutical market for diabetes drugs is more than 30 billion per year. This is a disease that was pretty rare a century ago. A new report by Visiongain predicts the world market for diabetes medications will reach $55.3bn in 2017. The anti-diabetic medicines industry generated $35.6bn in 2012, and its revenues will show strong growth to 2023. That sales forecast and others appear in Diabetes Treatments: World Drug Market 2013-2023, published in April 2013. Visiongain is a business information provider based in London, UK.

Everything we've been told about food and healthy eating by our governments and many paid off "scientists" has been wrong.

Developing an awareness of the foods you eat and learning how to read labels will help you make lifelong changes.

Naturally-occurring sugars, such as those in an apple or a pear, are not included in the less-than-10-percent-a-day recommendation because they are considered whole food. These affect your body completely different because they are packed with fiber and other nutrients.  You also don't have to watch your food intake with these sugars – except as part of your overall calories. If you are following a Keto lifestyle the best Low GI fruits are berries (such as raspberries, blueberries, strawberries and blackberries) in small amounts can allow you to stay in ketosis while still getting your fruit fix. Here are the carb and fiber counts for berries (per 1 cup serving): Blackberries:

14g of total carbs, 7g of sugar, 8g of fiber and 6g of net carbs.

You also have to watch out for added sugars – This is the sugar that you add to your food or beverage. Added sugars come in many different forms such as: Raw sugar, brown sugar, cane sugar, sucrose, glucose, fructose, malt, maltose, corn syrup, lactose, sorbitol, mannitol, honey, molasses, evaporated cane juice, and barley malt extract.

# Our Food Pyramid Is a Corrupt Foundation:
# It's All a BIG FAT Lie

More than 29 million adults in the U.S. — about 9 percent of the population — currently have diabetes, according to the Centers for Disease Control and Prevention. The obesity rate has more than doubled since 1980 and now hovers between 31 percent and 35 percent. About a half-million Americans die of heart disease every year, accounting for one in every four deaths.

Congress and the USDA has a HUGE interest in intentionally deceiving Americans into us believing that if we eat by their standards of the food pyramid that they created we will be healthy. In-fact this is far from the truth. The food pyramid was created by the USDA- (United States Department of Agriculture) to support modern industrial agriculture.  Follow the money. Congress has legislated nutrition labels to benefit large corporate donors. In 2011, congress blocked an attempt by the USDA to revise the school lunch program. Thanks to multi-million-dollar lobbing efforts by large food companies like Schwan's and Con-Agra foods, congress was able to protect the status quo for those companies. The status quo being that pizza sauce counts as a vegetable. No joke. Pizza sauce is considered a vegetable according to the US Congress. And here's the link to back it up.  NYTIMES – Congress Blocks New Rules on School Lunches

You see Minnesota's Schwan Food Co., is the country's largest supplier of school lunch pizzas.

To be fair the company responded to this by saying: "Schwan's has not, and does not, advocate that pizza replace the vegetable component of a balanced school meal," the company said in statement. "We are advocating that tomato paste — one tablespoon of which provides the equivalent nutrients of approximately three tomatoes —

continue to be credited for the nutrients it contains."

I am not debating the claim that tomato sauce will provide nutrients of approximately three tomatoes. What I have an issue with is the "extra" ingredients that are added.

This is an economic pushing for an industry that was designed by our government as a weapon and as a way to make profits and to do that they need customers. We are the customers and they also have taken over the FDA (The U.S. Food and Drug Administration).

Our taste buds have been hijacked by fake foods.

Part of the answer lies in the economics of the food industry: the profit margins and scale of money from processed food companies offer where the growers of healthy foods can't match.

In 2015, according to the Center for Responsive Politics, processed food manufacturers spent $32 million on lobbying while the fruit and vegetable industry spent a mere $3.7 million.

Follow the money. Kellogg's has a $26 billion market capitalization because it does not just make cereal. It also owns Pringles and manufactures a variety of processed foods from Eggo Waffles to Famous Amos chocolate chip cookies.

The entire processed foods industry is similarly consolidated. If you follow your favorite snack up the food chain, you'll usually find that it is owned by a multinational company. PepsiCo owns Funyuns, Rold Gold pretzels, and Sun Chips. Ritz crackers, Oreos, and Wheat Thins sell under the Nabisco label, which is owned by Mondelēz International. So whenever a federal agency supports healthy foods, it picks a fight with a collection of the world's largest companies.

It's a very simple logic: Supply and demand. If you have a demand for something, someone is going to supply you with it.

Again, everything we've been told about food and healthy eating by our governments and many paid off "scientists" has been wrong.

The USDA released their first set of nutrition guidelines in 1894.

A 2nd revision came out in 1943 which the USDA gave us the BASIC 7.

# For Health...eat some food from each group...every day!

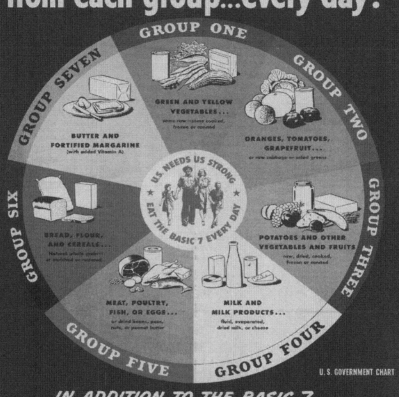

U.S. GOVERNMENT CHART

IN ADDITION TO THE BASIC 7...
EAT ANY OTHER FOODS YOU WANT

U.S. DEPARTMENT OF AGRICULTURE

In 1956, the USDA decided that there were actually only 4 food groups, and revised their nutrition yet again and those 4 food groups looked like this:

1. Vegetables and Fruits – This makes no sense. Fruits and vegetables do not fit the same dietary role.

2. Milk and Dairy.

3. Meat and proteins –

4. Cereals and Breads –

No mention of fats and we know that they are critical to body growth and function then there is #4 which is pretty much anything made from grains.

Healthy Dietary fat is required for proper hormone production and function. Also a diet rich in healthy fats like avocados, grass-fed butter, wild-caught salmon and coconut oil is associated with a lower risk of developing obesity.  This is just few of the many roles good healthy fats have in our body and why low-fat diets can be problematic for optimal health.

The "war on fat," is now coming to an end.

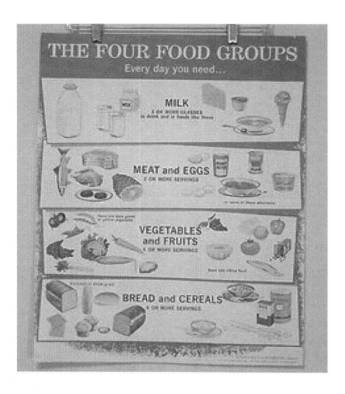

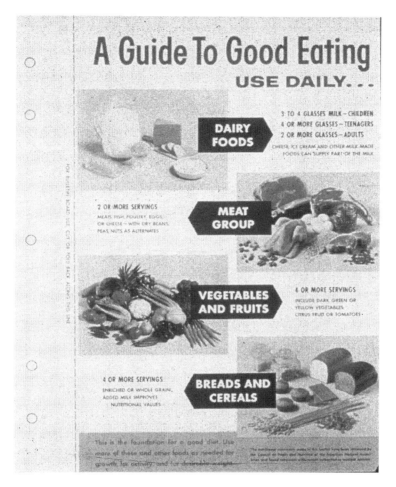

In 1961, another food guide line was issued after the scare of President Eisenhower had a heart attack. No one knew why, what, when or how heart disease occurs. Ancel Keys an American physiologist from the University of Minnesota, who studied the influence of diet on health. In particular, he hypothesized was that dietary saturated fat caused cardiovascular heart disease and should be avoided. He stated that saturated fats and cholesterol caused heart disease. Billions of dollars were spent to prove his hypothesis to be correct. He did a case study in seven different countries that he obviously cherry picked which ones to study. You see he started out with 22 countries and just tossed out the ones that didn't fit his hypothesis. After Keys deleted the countries who didn't fit his hypothesis, this only left him with only Japan, Italy, Great Britain, Australia, Canada and the US.

In 1992, the USDA came out with a new Food Pyramid.  Unlike the others this one states how healthy diet is breads, cereals, and other products made from grains. The government's "food pyramid" resulted in a dramatic rise in obesity, diabetes, cancer, and heart disease among other health issues.

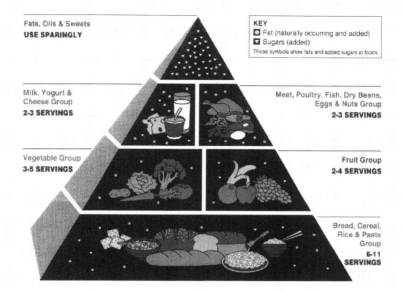

Fats, Oils & Sweets
**USE SPARINGLY**

KEY
◻ Fat (naturally occurring and added)
◪ Sugars (added)
These symbols show fats and added sugars in foods.

Milk, Yogurt &
Cheese Group
**2-3 SERVINGS**

Meat, Poultry. Fish, Dry Beans,
Eggs & Nuts Group
**2-3 SERVINGS**

Vegetable Group
**3-5 SERVINGS**

Fruit Group
**2-4 SERVINGS**

Bread, Cereal,
Rice & Pasta
Group
**6-11
SERVINGS**

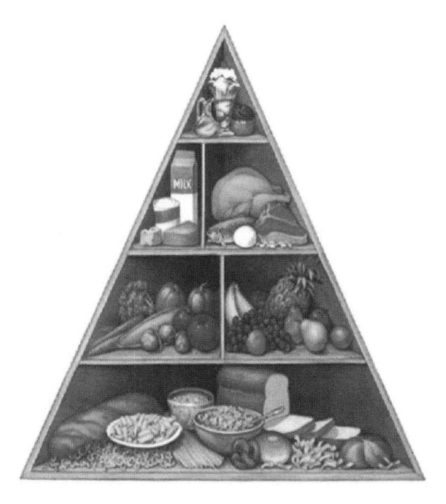

The government's "food pyramid" resulted in a dramatic rise in obesity, diabetes, and heart disease, among other health issues.

The bread you're buying at the store really isn't real bread you're buying. The white bread in the grocery is not the bread that our ancestors use to eat.  65% of the foods we eat are made from grains that are grown in a field such as grain bread, whiskey pasta and beer just to name a few. Wheat is made up of 3 parts the bran, the germ and the starchy endosperm.

The way the grain is processed has a huge impact not only on the way it tastes and how healthy it is for you. Our ancestors used every part of the grain when they made their bread. White bread on the store shelves is made by an industrial process that strips out the wheat into all-purpose flour and in most cases if you read the back of the labels you will see chemicals additives added. These chemical additives are what gives white bread a longer shelve life. White bread is also only made from the starchy endosperm which your body turns into pure sugar.

Yet again, it has been revised! This time they are suggesting cutting down on grains and increasing the amount of veggies recommended but what they fail to mention is to eat ORGANIC! Although you may eat more veggies which is always a great choice for your health, it's very vital to understand that many vegetables contain high levels of pesticides. A new analysis by the USDA actually revealed at least 34 unapproved pesticides on cilantro samples.

The Environmental Protection Agency (EPA) considers 60 percent of herbicides, 90 percent of fungicides, and 30 percent of insecticides to be carcinogenic, and most are damaging to your nervous system as well. In fact, these powerful and dangerous chemicals have been linked to numerous health problems such as:

Neurotoxicity and Parkinson's disease

Disruption of your endocrine system

Carcinogenicity

Immune system suppression

Miscarriages, male infertility and reduced reproductive function

This information should make you rethink when you are considering whether to buy local, organic vegetables or not.

Non-organic, un-rinsed vegetables are, first and foremost, grown with the use of toxic petrochemicals such as pesticides, herbicides, and just recently, antimicrobials as well. Residues of petrochemicals which have been directly sprayed onto the vegetables then remain on the outer leaves and skins of vegetables, though traces of them may be removed by thorough washing. Pesticide exposure has manifold detrimental side effects in humans

Now, with all this being said we can certainly begin to understand America's food industry and its lobbying process and we can begin to understand a certain mystery behind the food pyramid: why it was created and still promotes a diet although it certainly doesn't benefit the American people. Our Food Pyramid is Corrupt Foundation that can be bought.  There is so much more at stake here like wealth, power and social status.

If you take the current food pyramid and turn it upside-down that is what our food pyramid should look like. There's a lot of money to be made selling obesity foods, and you can't move America in a healthier direction without confronting the salty, sugary, and finger-licking, just-one-more-chip financial firepower of the food industrial complex.  "Good advice about nutrition conflicts with the interests of many big industries," Michael Jacobson, co-founder of the Center for Science in the Public Interest, has said, "each of which has more lobbying power than all the public-interest groups combined." But the real problem is that manufacturers of unhealthy food are so powerful that those interest's groups are always the pushing snack foods rather than fruit.

Our bodies have no way of adapting to these GMO and food like substances that we've been consuming. Every cell in your body is wrapped in a membrane of half fat and half protein. If you are constantly feeding these cells unnatural fatty acids, that membrane cannot function like it is designed to do and disease starts at the cellular level.

Dr. Luise Light is a nutrition expert and led the team at the Department of Agriculture that made the original recommendations for the food pyramid. If you review her original recommendations, they sound similar to dietary advice given by nutritionists today: lots of vegetables, more lean sources of protein like fish and nuts, and less dairy and processed foods.

Those guidelines, according to Dr. Light, did not survive their trip to the office of the Head of the Department of Agriculture. She has described herself as "shocked" by the changes that were made. Her team placed fruits and vegetables at the base of the pyramid and whole-grain breads and cereals further up. The new guidelines not only switched carbohydrates to the base of the pyramid, they moved processed foods like crackers and corn flakes, which Dr. Light and her team had placed at the top of the pyramid with chocolate, to the base too. Even with all the edits, the food pyramid was not released for another 12 years.

The American government has massive influence over our diet. Federal policy shapes our farm system to an astonishing level and this also is the reason why our unhealthy school lunch menu remains for millions of schoolchildren.

"Good advice about nutrition conflicts with the interests of many big industries," Michael Jacobson, co-founder of the Center for Science in the Public Interest, has said, "each of which has more lobbying power than all the public-interest groups combined." But the real problem is that manufacturers of unhealthy food are so powerful that those interest's groups are always the pushing snack foods rather than fruit.

There's a lot of money to be made selling obesity foods, and you can't move America in a healthier direction without confronting the salty, sugary, and finger-licking, just-one-more-chip financial firepower of the food industrial complex.

If you take the current food pyramid and turn it upside-down that is what our food pyramid should look like.


Looking at the bigger picture. Follow the money. It's a revolving door. This is bigger than any of us can imagine. It's more than just being lied to about the food pyramid. This revolving door certainly enables certain private vested interests to have a strong influence, way beyond that of us ordinary citizens, on how the government works, and that the country is still increasingly being run by a cozy group of insiders with ties to both government and industry.  Most people keep a blind eye to it and actually it's safer to not fight this fight or suggest anything alone these lines if you want to stay alive.  This has been termed crony capitalism. People have been killed for lesser whistle blower statements.

# Cleaning and Body Products
# Are
# Damaging Women's Health

The Environmental Protection Agency (EPA) suggests that:

Cleaning products are necessary for maintaining attractive and healthful conditions in the home and workplace. In addition to the obvious aesthetic benefits of cleaning, the removal of dust, allergens, and infectious agents is crucial to maintaining a healthful indoor environment.

The real reality is we are damaging our DNA and we are changing our genetic makeup for future generations. There was a study a few years back that said the umbilical cord of an average American baby has over 200 known chemicals in it. Eighty percent of the common chemicals that are used daily in this country, we know almost nothing about. Our children are being born toxic and we have no idea if these toxins are already doing some sort of damage their brains, their immune system, their reproductive system, and any other developing organs. Are we unknowingly setting ourselves up for failure in the womb, even before birth?

Scientists and researchers are concerned that many of these chemicals may be carcinogenic or wreak havoc with our hormones, our body's regulating system. But the impact of these chemicals may be most severe on the developing brain, Perera said.

Brain development is the "most complete and most rapid during the first nine months, prenatally," she said. During that time, neural connections and pathways are being developed.

"Any interference by a physical stress like a toxic chemical or other stressor can disrupt this natural progression that is so very delicate and complex," explained Perera.

Though the group hopes to come up with regulatory recommendations to reduce this toxic burden, there are some simple things that individuals can do to reduce their exposure.

Children exposed to higher levels of these pesticides have been found to have higher rates of attention-deficit hyperactivity disorder.

Most products have a warning label that is typed in bold "Keep out of Reach of Children". As consumers, we believe that if our children don't ingest these products they will not be harmed by them. This can be far from the truth. Think about other common methods of exposure are through the skin and our respiratory tract. WE are along with our children are often in contact with the chemical residues housecleaning products do leave behind, by crawling, lying and sitting on the freshly cleaned floor.

Scientists at Norway's University of Bergen tracked 6,000 people, with an average age of 34 at the time of enrollment in the study, who used the cleaning products over a period of two decades, according to the research published in the American Thoracic Society's American Journal of Respiratory and Critical Care Medicine.

They found that lung function decline in women who regularly used the products, such as those who worked as cleaners, was equivalent over the period to those with a 20-cigarette daily smoking habit.

Everyday chemicals carry toxic burden

These chemicals can chemicals bind together.

Exposure to phthalates has been associated with lower IQ levels.

These chemicals can also be found in the shampoos, conditioners, body sprays, hair sprays, perfumes, make up, cleaning supplies, colognes, soap and nail polish that we use.

The results follow a study by French scientists in September 2017 that found nurses who used disinfectants to clean surfaces at least once a week had a 24 percent to 32 percent increased risk of developing lung disease.

Scientists and researchers are concerned that many of these chemicals may be carcinogenic or wreak havoc with our hormones, our body's regulating system.

It's not enough to be aware of all the outdoor chemicals that we are exposed to everyday but inside our homes we can have more power and control. We have to be more aware about using chemical cleaners, paints, glues, body lotions, toothpastes, underarm deodorants, hair products and pesticides. Instead start to begin to use products that don't pollute our very own bodies. We must read labels, make our own products and do our own research. I can't stress this enough. We must take a stand for our health. Stop using commercial products that are laced with unknown and harmful body damaging products.

Did you know that products we use every day may contain toxic chemicals and has been linked to women's health issues? They are hidden endocrine disruptors and are very tricky chemicals that play havoc on our bodies. "We are all routinely exposed to endocrine disruptors, and this has the potential to significantly harm the health of our youth," said Renee Sharp, EWG's director of research. "It's important to do what we can to avoid them, but at the same time we can't shop our way out of the problem. We need to have a real chemical policy reform." The longer the length of ingredients on your food label means how much more unhealthy it is for you to consume. When an item contains a host of ingredients that most likely you can't even pronounce or remember to spell you can bet your lucky dollar that the natural nutrients are long gone. These highly processed frank "n" foods are very difficult for the body to break down and some of the chemicals will become stored in your body. Click on this link to see what you should avoid.

Pesticides, herbicides, GMOs in our food, fluoride and chlorine and trace pharmaceutical residue in the water supplies, methane, carbon monoxide and industrial pollutants in the air, and the toxic chemicals in our everyday household products.

No wonder our bodies are completely bombarded and overwhelmed with the constant exposed to toxic chemicals through the air that we breathe, the water we drink, the foods we eat, and the personal care products and cleaning products we use.

Every Cell in your body responds to the foods you eat, the products you put on your body to the house hold chemicals that you purchase for your home. All of these things have a direct impact on your hormones and in return your hormones have a direct impact on every major system in your body. Not to mention that our body is lacking certain nutrients that heavily influence the function of every cell in our body.

For starters, the three essential categories into which most of the hazardous ingredients in household cleaning products fall are:

1. Carcinogens– Carcinogens cause cancer and/or promote cancer's growth.

2. Endocrine disruptors – Endocrine disruptors mimic human hormones, confusing the body with false signals. Exposure to endocrine disruptors can lead to numerous health concerns including reproductive, developmental, growth and behavior problems. Endocrine disruptors have been linked to reduced fertility, premature puberty, miscarriage, menstrual problems, challenged immune systems, abnormal prostate size, ADHD, non-Hodgkin's lymphoma and certain cancers.

3. Neurotoxins – Neurotoxins alter neurons, affecting brain activity, causing a range of problems from headaches to loss of intellect

## TAKING CUES FROM PRODUCT LABELS

You may find it time-consuming to research all of the ingredients in the cleaning products under the kitchen sink, in your garage or even in the bathroom but trust me. It is worth the hassle. Over all, product warning labels can be a useful first line of defense. These companies are required by law to include label warnings on their cleaning products if harmful ingredients are included. From safest to most dangerous, the warning signals are:

Signal Word

Toxicity if swallowed, inhaled or absorbed through the skin*

Caution

One ounce to a pint may be harmful or fatal

Warning

One teaspoon to one ounce may be harmful or fatal

Danger

One taste to one teaspoon is fatal


The diagnosis and treatment of thyroid disease has nearly failed nearly 59 million people. Our bodies are completely bombarded and overwhelmed with the constant exposed to toxic chemicals through the air that we breathe, the water we drink, the foods we eat, personal care products and cleaning products we use.

What happens when you combine fast food, toxic vaccines, flu shots, fluoride-loaded tap water, pesticides and dangerous, chemical-based prescription medications? Nobody really knows. There has never been a study on the effects of how combing all these things on a daily basis does to our body.

People are using products on their body and in their homes and that are hormone disruptors. No one can force you to become more aware of what you put on your body and what you put in your body. What you eat is just as important as what you put on your body. Adjusting your life, reading labels and catering to your specific health needs isn't easy but it will benefit you in the long run. This is one of the smartest decisions that you can make. Not only will you start to look and feel better but think of the medical cost that you could be saving your future self.

Those pesky endocrine disruptors that I keep mentioning have tricky chemicals in them that play on our bodies. They increase production of certain hormones; decreasing production of others; imitating hormones; turning one hormone into another; interfering with hormone signaling; telling cells to die prematurely; competing with essential nutrients; binding to essential hormones; accumulating in organs that produce hormones. You can start avoiding these chemicals by starting with detoxifying your home and beauty products.


DIY Liquid Hand Soap

   1/2 cup Dr. Bronners Liquid Castile Soap

   1/2 cup distilled water

   1 TB vitamin E oil (optional)

   1 TB sweet almond oil or olive oil or jojoba oil (optional)

   5 drops lemon essential oil

   5 drops lavender essential oil

   In a Mason jar or recycled soap dispenser, add the water first (to prevent bubbles) then the liquid castile soap, followed by the oils. Shake the ingredients together.

   Shake the soap dispenser before using, then squirt a small amount on your hands as needed, rinsing with water.

# Natural Citrus Antibacterial Liquid Hand Soap

1/2 cup Dr. Bonners Liquid Castile Soap

1/2 cup distilled water

1 TB vitamin E oil

1 TB sweet almond oil, apricot kernel oil, olive oil or jojoba oil

5 drops lemon essential oil

5 drops On Guard essential oil

In a Mason jar or recycled soap dispenser, add the water first (to prevent bubbles) then the liquid castile soap, followed by the oils. Shake the ingredients together.

Shake the soap dispenser before using, then squirt a small amount on your hands as needed, rinsing with water.

Mosquito Repellent

15 drops of lavender

4 tbsp. of vanilla extract

1/4 cup freshly squeezed lemon juice

Place all these ingredients in a 16oz then fill with water.


Bathroom Cleaner

3 tsp baking soda

1 TBSP of washing soda (optional)

8 oz. very hot water

1 TBSP Sal Suds

About 1 cup room temperature water

$\frac{1}{4}$ tsp lemon essential oil

$\frac{1}{2}$ tsp orange essential oil

10 drops cinnamon leaf essential oil

$\frac{1}{4}$ tsp clove essential oil

OR 1 tsp of a "thieves" essential oil instead of these other blends

16 oz. glass spray bottle

Pour the baking soda, washing soda and hot water in the spray bottle, then the hot water. Close the lid on the bottle, and shake well until the powder dissolves. Remove the cap and then add the Sal Suds and essential oils. Fill the remainder of the bottle with water until the bottle is almost full, making sure to leave room for the sprayer lid. Give it another shake to combine the mixture and spray on the area you want to clean. Always use a clean cloth or sponge when cleaning.

Hard water Stain Remover

1 cup of Epsom salt

1/2 cup of baking soda

1/4 cup of Sal suds

$\frac{1}{2}$ cup warm water

Pour the warm water into the bottle, followed by the baking soda and Epsom salt. Shake the bottle to combine the ingredients. Add the Sal suds gently shaking the bottle to combine. Scrub and then rinse with water and wet clean rag.


Soap scum and residue cleaner

    1 1/2 cups baking soda

    1/2 cup natural liquid castile soap

    1/2 cup water

    2 tablespoons distilled white vinegar

Pour the warm water into the bottle, followed by the baking soda and Epsom salt. Shake the bottle to combine the ingredients. Add the Sal suds gently shaking the bottle to combine. Put a small amount of this mixture onto a sponge, wash the surface, and then rinse well.

Non-abrasive soft scrubber

   1/4 cup baking soda

   1 teaspoon liquid castile soap or Sal Suds

   1/2 teaspoon lemon essential oil

Mix the baking soda with just enough soap to form a creamy paste. Add the lemon oil and combine well. Put a small amount of this mixture onto a sponge, wash the surface, and then rinse well.


Toilet Bowl Cleaner with hydrogen peroxide

      1/4 to 1/2 cup Hydrogen Peroxide

   1 cup Baking Soda

   3 – 5 drops Essential Oils (Lemon, Lavender, Tea Tree, thieves or Clove are great choices to disinfect and freshen the air)

1/2 cup castile soap

Sprinkle all ingredients around the toilet bowl; hydrogen peroxide first, then baking soda, last the essential oil. Allow it to sit for 15 minutes. Scrub and then rinse well

## Bathroom Mold disinfecting spray

You don't have to grab bleach to get rid of mold in your bathroom. This 3 combo all natural mixture will do the trick. I will spray the areas in my bathroom and leave it on for 10 minutes and wipe the moldy areas away. Vodka might be a little bit pricey but you won't be breathing in toxic chemicals or having to worry about your skin absorbing a list of toxic chemicals. Vinegar is naturally antimicrobial, tea tree is natural fungicide which can eliminate any mold or mildew problems and kills black mold spores! Don't forget to label your spray bottle with a black permanent marker.

1 cup of white vinegar

1 cup of vodka

10 drops of tea tree oil

No need to dilute any of this mixture. Place all the ingredients in a spray bottle and label it bathroom mold killer. Mix well. Spray onto hard surfaces where mold and mildew are growing and let this amazing combo do its cleaning. You'll still have to scrub a bit, but with repeated use this all-natural cleaner will kill the fungus and help to prevent future growth. Shake each time before use.

Homemade powder laundry soap

   2/3 cup Super-Washing Soda

   3 tbsp. Baking Soda

   $\frac{1}{2}$ cup Liquid Castile soap

5 cups of water, divided

Directions

   Bring 5 cups of water to a boil.

   Pour washing soda into a large glass bowl then slowly stir in 2 cups of boiling water until washing soda is completely dissolved. Don't forget to label with a black permanent marker.

## Easy Floor cleaner

1 cup of white vinegar

1 tablespoon of Sal Suds or dawn detergent as shown in the photo

1 cup of baking soda

2 gallons of very warm water

Mix in a bucket and always use a clean mop.

## Natural Counter Disinfectant Spray

This natural disinfectant can clean germs that cause food borne illness on your kitchen counter tops. Tea tree oil is a naturally-occurring essential oil with anti-fungal properties that can kill staphylococcus, e-coli and salmonella. The vinegar has acid qualities that also help to kill germs and reduce microbial growth. The castile soap gives it an extra cleansing boost.  Make sure to not spray this on or near your food.

2 cups of water

20 drops of lemon essential oil or tea tree oil

1 cup white distilled vinegar

1 tsp Dr. Bonner's liquid castile soap

Fill your bottle with water, drop in the tea tree oil and next add the vinegar. Seal the lid, give it a good shake then lastly add your castile soap. Place the sprayer on the bottle, seal tightly and shake. You can label your bottle with a black magic marker: Kitchen Cleaner. This recipe can be used with tea tree oil in place of the lemon but I prefer not to because tea tree oil can be toxic to pets that is why I use lemon. Don't forget to label your spray bottle with a black permanent marker.

Tub & Tile Cleaner

1 /4 cup baking soda

1/4 cup lemon juice

Or 10 drops of lemon essential oil

3 Tablespoons Epsom salt

3 Tablespoons Sal Suds or Castile liquid soap

1/2 cup white vinegar

Pour the vinegar into the bottle, followed by the baking soda and Epsom salt. Shake the bottle to combine the ingredients. Add the Sal suds gently shaking the bottle to combine. Mix all ingredients in a bottle with a sealable lid.

Scrub and then rinse with water and wet clean rag.


Vanilla grapefruit linen spray

2-1/2 cups filtered water

3 drops pink grapefruit essential oil

2 drops vanilla essential oil

1/4 cup vodka

The vodka helps the water dry quickly after you spray it on your linens. Theses essential oils that are used create a beautifully fresh vanilla grapefruit scent that is perfect for a summer pick me up. This spray is very versatile. It can be used on clothing, fabric furniture, or even as a quick air freshener.

If the vodka smell is slightly strong just add another drop or two of essential oil.

Always shake the bottle be before spraying on your linen.


Taking a soaking hot bath 2x a week for 20 minutes each is very beneficial! It can help to draws out toxins, helps to lower stress related hormones and assists in balancing your ph levels.


Epsom salt bath which is rich in magnesium

Sleepy time Goats Milk Bath

2 cups of powdered goat's milk

2 cup of Epsom salt

1 cup of sea salt

2 cup of baking soda

10 drops of lavender essential oil

Combine the dry ingredients and the lavender essential oil. Store in a closed container. When you are ready to take a bath add 1 cup of dry ingredients. (Kids can use up to 1/2 cup of the mixture). Bathe 3 times weekly, soaking for at least 12 minutes.


Nourishing Homemade Body Wash

   1/2 cup full-fat unsweetened coconut milk canned

   2/3 cup Dr. Bonner's lavender Liquid Castile Soap

   3 tsp vitamin E oil

5 drops lavender essential oil

2 tablespoons jojoba, apricot kernel oil, almond oil, or olive oil

Combine all ingredients in a bottle or Mason jar with a sealable lid. When you want to use it just shake the container and pour on a washcloth. This body wash doesn't have any preservatives and it contains coconut milk therefore it has a short lifespan. I keep this in my fridge and use it within a week.


DIY Skin Smoother Detox Bath

2 cups Epsom salt

2 cups baking soda

2 cups sea salt

1 cup vinegar

$\frac{1}{4}$ cup of organic coconut oil (this will melt in the hot bath)

Directions: combine the dry ingredients, store in a closed container.  When you are ready to take a bath add 1 cup of dry ingredients, 1 cup of vinegar and ¼ cup of coconut oil.   (Kids can use up to a 1/2 cup of the mixture). Bathe 3 times weekly, soaking for at least 12 minutes.

## Shampoo

¼ cup canned coconut milk

1/4 cup Dr. Bonners Liquid Castile Soap

20 drops of Essential Oils of choice

For dry hair: add ½ tsp olive or almond oil

Pour all the ingredients in an old shampoo bottle or Mason jar with some kind (pump soap dispensers and even foaming dispensers work well for this. If you use a foaming dispenser, add 1/4 cup of distilled water) Make sure to shake well before each use and this will keep for about a month in your shower. I use about a teaspoon every time I shampoo my hair.

This also can be used as a shaving cream but just dilute it with 1/4 cup distilled water.

Rosemary Honey Conditioner

16 oz. of local, raw or Manuka honey

10 drops of rosemary essential oil

Mix the Rosemary essential oil & honey in a mason or bowl. I use about 1 tablespoon at of time of the honey mixture. I just place it in my hands and spread on my hair. Make sure your hair is completely wet because his is very sticky and you want to be able to lather is around all over your head.

Rose water Hair Perfume

In a 4oz glass spray bottle add 1 teaspoon pure vanilla extract with 3 drops of the essential oil of your choice and fill to the top of the bottle with rosewater. Spritz on your hair as it is drying and style as usual. Store in the refrigerator for several weeks.

# How to Make Rose Water

1/4 cup of dried organic, pesticide-free rose petals

1 1/2 cups water

Pour 1 1/2 cups water into your stockpot and add the rose petals. Bring the petals to a boil then turn down the stove to allow it to simmer for 10 minutes. Remove from the hot eye and place a lid on the pot. Allow the water to completely cool. Once it has completely cooled. Pour water and petals through a nut bag or cheesecloth into a dark, clean bottle. You can place the rose water in the refrigerator for several weeks or on the counter for up to one week.

# Shear hand Lotion

- 1 cup pure shea butter
- 1 cup pure coconut oil
- 1/3 cup arrowroot powder
- 2 tsp melted beeswax pastilles
- 25 drops of lavender essential oil

Or you can also try out these other essential oil combinations:

5 drops eucalyptus and 5 drops spearmint

5 drops fir and 5 drops grapefruit

4 drops orange, 3 drops cedar wood, and 2 drops ylang ylang

3 drops patchouli and 6 drops tangerine

5 drops lavender and 5 drops lemon

Over low heat in a double boiler, put the coconut oil, shea butter and beeswax pastilles in a bowl. When it has almost completely melted, remove from the heat and add the arrowroot powder and essential oil.

Mix well and allow the mixture to cool until it solidifies. Lastly mix the body butter vigorously with a spatula until soft peaks form, and then transfer it to a mason jar with a sealable lid. Date and label your product.

Homemade "Vaseline"

Ingredients

1/4 cup coconut oil

1/8 cup olive oil

2 tablespoons beeswax

2 drops peppermint essential oil (optional or your favorite smell)

Over medium heat you want to melt the coconut oil and beeswax to combine. After its melted remove from the heat, pour in the EVOO and mix the ingredients together. Allow it to cool but you want it still pourable so you can pour the mixture into a mason jar and add your essential oil which is optional.  This homemade Vaseline will keep fresh on the counter for up to a year.

Homemade Calamine Lotion

All the ingredients in this homemade Calamine lotion are safe and effective.

Bentonite clay: will help bind to the oils from the Poison Ivy plant and     helps reduce the itchiness

Baking soda: will neutralize the acid and soothes the itch

Sea salt: will reduce the inflammation and also help dry out the oils

Glycerin: this will give your lotion a smooth consistency and help for a nice glide

1/8 cup water

4 tsps. Natural Calcium Bentonite Clay

4 tsps. Baking Soda

1 Tbsp. Celtic Sea Salt

1 tsp Glycerin (optional)

In a bowl mix all the dry ingredients until well combined. Add the water and mix until you get the desired consistency (you might need more or less water). Next add in the glycerin (this will give your lotion a smooth consistency, for a nice glide) lastly, place lotion in a mason jar with a sealable lid. Date and label the lid.


Calming Magnesium Body Butter

   1/2 cup cocoa butter

   1/2 cup of coconut oil and melt

   1/4 cup magnesium oil

Add 10 drops of lavender essential oil,

 Add 10 drops cedarwood essential oil

  Add 10 drops frankincense essential oil

Place a heat-safe glass measuring cup/bowl inside a pot that has 1-2 inches of simmering water over medium heat. Add the cocoa butter and melt it in your double boiler until it's completely melted.

Remove the cocoa butter from heat, and add 1/2 cup extra virgin coconut oil to the melted cocoa butter and stir until completely the coconut oil has melted. Next add 1/4 cup magnesium oil to the mixture and combine. Place the mixture in the refrigerator to cool for about 30-60 minutes (until it is cooled completely). After the mixture has completely cooled and became a solid. Use a hand mixer or stand mixer to whip it. Start on low and increase speed slowly. Whip for about 3-5 minutes. Next add the 10 drops each of lavender essential oil, the 10 drops of cedar wood essential oil, and the 10 drops of frankincense essential oil. Scrape down the sides of the bowl and continue whipping for another 5 minutes or so, until the magnesium body butter is light and fluffy.

The color of the magnesium body butter will change from yellow to a pale ivory and almost white color. Lastly put the magnesium body butter into mason jars and seal tightly with a lid. Make sure to label and date the top of the lid. This recipe makes enough for two 4 oz. glass jars.

## Homemade Lip Balm - with Tint

2 tbsp. beeswax

2 tbsp. coconut oil

1/4-1/2 tsp vanilla extract

Beet root powder -

Place a heat-safe glass measuring cup/bowl inside a pot that has 1-2 inches of simmering water over medium heat. Add the beeswax & coconut oil.  Melt it in your double boiler until it's completely melted. Once the beeswax is melted, add the vanilla extract and lip color/beet root powder.  Stir. Pour into containers and allow to cool completely.

If you don't want tint leave out the beet root.

Lavender and Rose Water Toner

    4 tablespoons rose water

    2 tablespoons witch hazel

    1 teaspoon apple cider vinegar

    5-10 drops rosehip oil

    1 drop lavender oil or your favorite essential oil scent

In a small bowl, place the rose water, witch hazel, apple cider vinegar, rosehip oil, and lavender oil. Combine well and transfer to a small glass bottle. After you have cleansed your face, pour some on a cotton ball and rub over your face. Once it has dried add your favorite natural facial moisturizer.

# Anti-Aging Facial Toner

1/2 cup brewed and cooled green tea

1/4 cup witch hazel

2 drops citrus oil such as grapefruit

2 drops rosemary

3 drops frankincense

3 drops carrot seed

2 oz. glass spray bottles with fine mist sprayer

Brew the tea and place it in a cup along with the tea bag to sit overnight in the refrigerator. Pour 1/2 cup of green tea in a spray bottle, add 1/4 cup of witch hazel and the essential oils. Tightly close the lid on the bottle and shake vigorously. Mist-spray directly on face and pat with clean hands. The toner will dry quickly. Keep this toner in your refrigerator. You can also apply this with a small amount added to a cotton ball or pad.

Lemon Honey Face Mask

1 tsp fresh squeezed lemon juice

1 tsp local, raw or Manuka Honey

1-2 drops frankincense essential oil

Mix the ingredients until they become a liquid texture. Apply on a clean face and allow to sit for 20 minutes or longer. Rinse with warm water and apply moisturizer of your choice.

Lemon Cream Body Butter

This smells like summer.

6 Tablespoons coconut oil

$\frac{1}{4}$ cup cocoa butter

1 Tablespoon vitamin E oil

3 drops of Lemon essential oil or 3 drops of your favorite essential oil

Over low heat in a double boiler, put the coconut oil and cocoa butter in a bowl. When it has almost completely melted, remove from the heat and add the vitamin E oil and essential oil. Allow the mixture to cool until it solidifies. Lastly mix the body butter vigorously with a spatula, and then transfer it to a mason jar with a sealable lid. Date and label your product. If you don't care for the lemon essential oil, use whatever smells best to you. This is your journey not mine I am only here to help guide you.

Anti-wrinkle cream

5 drops of almond oil

1/8 slice of a fresh avocado

Place the ingredients in a bowl and mash with a fork. Combine well. Apply on your face with a brush gently or your fingertips. Rinse off, gently, after 1 hour.

I also like to keep my eye cream or facial cream in my fridge!

Always remember: Cold constricts, heat expands.

Homemade Shaving Cream

1 cup shea butter

1 cup virgin coconut oil

3 Tablespoons vitamin E oil

3 Tablespoons sweet almond oil or olive oil or jojoba oil

3 Tablespoons Dr. Bonners Liquid Castile Soap

30 drops of lavender essential oil (optional)

30 drops of lemon essential oil (optional)


I like to use an electric mixer, mixing all ingredients until stiff peaks are formed (approximately 2-3 minutes). Store in a mason jar with a sealable lid.

# Self-Sabotaging your Workouts

We all know that regular exercise is an important part of your overall health. Exercise burns calories to prevent weight gain and helps speed up your metabolism. It is also a releases endorphins to give you those mood-enhancing chemicals. What if I told you that exercise can cause adrenal crashes due to your already high cortisol issues? You could be stressing your thyroid out even more and not even realizing it. Are you exercising but not getting any results? Are you still gaining weight, feeling constantly fatigued, irritable and moody and often battling some other sort of sickness? You could be actually stressing your body more out by over-exercising.

# The magic word here is cortisol.

Cortisol, a steroid hormone produced by the adrenal gland. It is released in response to stress. When you are stressed, your body releases certain "fight-or-flight" stress hormones that are produced in the adrenal glands: cortisol, norepinephrine and epinephrine. Staying stressed raises your cortisol levels and your body actually resists weight loss. Your body thinks times are hard and you might starve, so it hoards the fat you eat or what you have presently on your body. Cortisol will grab fat from your butt and hips, and move it to your abdomen which has more cortisol receptors. Hello there Mrs. Muffin Top!

Today most of us are in a chronic stress state. However, our body don't know the difference between car troubles, relationship issues, debt, work pressure and truly life-threatening stress. This is why our body still ready to defend and reacts exactly the same as it always has done.

Over-exercising can:

Deplete hormones necessary for the functioning of the body

Cause gradual bone loss

Increase injuries

Cause cramping of muscles

Add to inflammation

Increase healing time

Affect cardiac function

Affect blood flow

Decrease the ability of muscles to use fatty acids as a source of energy

Reduce endurance

Here are a few things you can start to incorporate into your life:

1. Avoid caffeine

2. Start eating a true Keto AIP diet. In doing this you will avoid simple carbs, processed foods, and refined grains, and get plenty of high-quality protein, healthy fats and great vegetables.

3. It's okay to say NO! Take time to relax, take a nap, distress and recuperate.

4. Start building your endurance back slowly.

5. Get a heart rate monitor and use it. Know your heart rate comfort zone.

6. Listen to your body. How do you feel the next day? Do you need an extra day to recover?

7. Set realistic goals, one step at a time and don't get discouraged.

8.    Try a Low-impact aerobics workout. Something to get your heart rate up and your lungs going without putting too much

pressure on your joints, which is important because joint pain is another common hypothyroidism symptom.

9. Strength training is good.  Strength training builds muscle mass, and muscle burns more calories than fat, even when you're at rest.

10. Get some sleep!

Just think how great it's going to feel when you are as healthy on the inside as you look on the outside! The ultimate goal isn't to look fit but to be fit.

# Get some sleep!

If you're not getting enough rest it will cause your body to become suppressed, which will slow your body from healing itself. You need to have a healthy sleep cycle. Many reasons why you may suffer from insomnia, difficulty falling asleep or even staying asleep but nutritional imbalances, environmental toxins, stress, hormonal imbalances and thyroid issues all can play a role in your sleep cycle. You need to look at your life. Environmental factors, dietary habits, and medical history all play a role in this.

It's amazing how the food we eat affects our health, sleep patterns and even our "gasp" sex drives. Unfortunately, when you don't get enough sleep, it can age us faster , cause depression, weight gain, make us forget things, gives us headaches and we have a greater chance of developing heart disease.  If you have issues like snoring or sleep apnea and are overweight, one thing you can do is lower your body fat index. For those of us that don't have snoring or sleep apnea we ask the question," Sleep why you hate me so much!" We need to feed our bodies to get more, Tryptophan, serotonin and melatonin. (Serotonin is a brain chemical that helps you sleep) and melatonin (the hormone that makes you sleepy) Trytophan is an essential amino acid, which means you have to get it from your diet because your body cannot produce it. Your body uses tryptophan to make the neurotransmitters serotonin and melatonin.

It's all in your daily patterns and diet. Your choice, your lifestyle. Always check with your health care provider before starting a new regime.

# Tips to guide you to better sleep

Turn off the electronics! That hand held device that you've been glued to all day? You have to put it down if you want to get some sound sleep—and the same goes for your laptop and iPad, too. Why? The blue wavelengths produced by your smartphone and other gadgets (and energy-efficient LED light bulbs) significantly suppress the production of melatonin, the hormone that makes you sleepy, according to University of Basel research. Another problem: Light-emitting devices engage and stimulate the mind, resulting in poorer sleep, according to an Osaka University study.

Avoid large meals late in the evening.

Learn and use a relaxation technique regularly. Breathing exercises, meditation and yoga are good examples. EXERCISE early in the day!!

Use "white noise" devices to block out surrounding environmental noise.

Take a warm bath with Epsom salt at night before bed

*NO CAFFINE PRODUCTS AFTER NOON!*

Lower the room temperature

8oz of cherry juice (Cherry juice-according to researchers from the Universities of Pennsylvania and Rochester. Cherries, particularly tart cherries, naturally boost levels of melatonin. A 2011 study found that cherries may be a natural sleep aid because of their melatonin levels)

## Red Onion Tea

Helps with insomnia

Directions

1 cup of water

1 onion, cut in quarters

Blend, strain and drink


Epsom salt bath which is rich in magnesium

## Sleepy time Goats Milk Bath

2 cups of powdered goat's milk

2 cup of Epsom salt

1 cup of sea salt

2 cup of baking soda

10 drops of lavender essential oil

Combine the dry ingredients and the lavender essential oil. Store in a closed container. When you are ready to take a bath add 1 cup of dry ingredients. (Kids can use up to 1/2 cup of the mixture). Bathe 3 times weekly, soaking for at least 12 minutes.

Lavender has a reputation as a mild tranquilizer. Simply dab a bit of the oil onto your temples and forehead before you hit the pillow. The aroma should help send you off to sleep.

Lastly, don't obsess over not sleeping. Studies have shown that people who worry about falling asleep have greater trouble falling asleep! It may help to remind yourself that while sleeplessness is a pain in the ass it isn't life-threatening. Let's try to be mellow-bellow. Eat foods that foods contribute to calmness and sleepiness.

# 5 plants to help you sleep better!

1. Aloe Vera — emits oxygen at night to help you combat insomnia and improve the overall sleep quality.

2. Lavender- Lavender is a plant that is well known to induce sleep and reduce anxiety. The smell of lavender slows down your heart rate and reduces anxiety levels.

3. Jasmine plant- The smell of jasmine has been shown to improve the quality of sleep.

4. English Ivy- it's beneficial for those who have breathing problems and asthma. Studies have shown that English ivy can reduce air molds to 94% in 12 hours.

5. Snake plant- emits oxygen into the night while you sleep, taking carbon dioxide from the air inside your home. It also filters nasty household toxins from the home.

Just think how great it's going to feel when you are as healthy on the inside as you look on the outside! The ultimate goal isn't to look fit but to be fit.

Many people are unaware that certain foods are actually working against their bodies. If you are allergic to certain foods it will involve you're the immune system. The immune system controls how your body defends itself. Your body see's inflammatory foods as invaders and will kick in your autoimmunity responses. For example if you have a food allergy to cow's milk, your immune system will see cow's milk as an invader.

# Intermittent Fasting

I don't want to make your head spin and you don't have to fast but I wanted to explain what it was and how it worked. If you don't care to try it, please don't eat 3 hours prior to bedtime and give your body an 8-hour break from consuming any food unless its water or a decaf herbal tea. (Unless you have a pre-diagnosed medical condition where your doctor has stated otherwise)

I Love intermittent fasting because it gives my body a break from the hard work of digestion and allows it to begin to rebook itself naturally.

Let me explain more about intermittent fasting. It's a technique where a person allows their digestive system to rest without eating, usually for a time period of 12, 14, 16, or 18 hours and then they eat during the remaining time frame. The idea also is to eat the amount of calories that your body requires and healthy during your allotted eating time frame. You are not starving yourself or calorie restricting.

For example, if you were to do a 12-hour fast, you're eating window would be 12 hours. You could start your eating window at 7am and end at 7pm. By Intermittent fasting you won't eat anything 2-3 hours prior to bed. You would break the fast the next day at 7am.

This new fasting technique has been known to boost energy levels, regulates blood sugar, improve weight-loss, increase motivation, better absorption of nutrients, stamina, along with improve cognitive function and it also will release the growth hormone that helps to repair your body. There are studies documenting showing many benefits of fasting which are can be lowering the risk of type 2 diabetes, reducing cholesterol levels, enhancing the body's resistance to oxidative stress (which is connected to aging and many chronic diseases), reducing your inflammation and of course weight loss!

Our hormonal balance is very sensitive to how much we eat, how often we eat, and what we eat. By calories restricting and over exercising (creating more cortisol; cortisol collects in your belly area) it will send a hormonal stress signal to your body and If the Intermittent fasting isn't done correctly it will also send a threat signal to a women's reproductive system and in return send a threat signal to your metabolism, ultimately slowing it down. Putting your body in a safe starvation mode where it can stay alive.

Therefore, you must eat what your body requires calorie wise and healthy to fuel it but let me be very clear this isn't for everyone because we are all created differently and like I mentioned before you may have a pre-diagnosed medical condition that your doctor advises against intermittent fasting.

During an IF you also can experience other symptoms, such as:

Sleeplessness

Anxiety

Irregular periods

Hormone dysregulation

Brain fog

You must understand that the female reproductive system and metabolism are deeply intertwined among each other. You see women store healthy fat for the chance they may become pregnant. Believe or not but pregnancy is the ultimate goal from an evolutionary perspective to keep humans from going extinct. Yes, you might not be trying or you might be done with your baby maker but if your still ovulating, your body isn't. You see without an ample amount of fat stored in your body that only can mean malnutrition for the future baby and possibility death to the fetus since your body wouldn't be able to sustain life.

A Women's body is very sensitive to anything that might signal starvation. If you are not eating enough calories or getting the right nutrients your body will produce more hunger hormones called leptin and ghrelin. Your body actually needs calories to burn calories and by restricting calories it will certainly backfire and throw your body into "starvation mode where it will actually slow down your metabolism, making it tougher for you to lose weight. I know, it sounds a bit complicated but no one is created equal and if you already have hypothyroidism or hormonal issues going on why throw fuel on the fire? Therefore it is very important that you feed your body the proper caloric intake. Even if you decide not to try Intermittent Fasting feeding your body notorious fats, low GI high fiber organic vegetables and clean high quality proteins are vital. Until you become Keto AIP-adapted you might have to add healthy fats like for example adding extra avocado oil to your salads.

Did you really read what I just wrote?

Your body actually needs calories to burn calories and by restricting calories it will certainly backfire and throw your body into "starvation mode" where it will actually slow down your metabolism, making it tougher for you to lose weight. I am certainly guilty of going through a phrase in my life where I only eating once a day thinking this was your solution. Oh How I was so very wrong! I was making myself fatter by not eating! Your body is trying to survive. You must eat to let your body know that it is its okay to burn those calories instead of storing them as fat.

Do you notice that when you become stressed you seem to crave fatty or salty foods? It means that your adrenals have become taxed from being overly stressed. Feed your body what it needs, listen to it but feed it good fats.

We must work with our bodies and not against it. We must always listen to our bodies, and realize that you are fierce piece of optimal machinery and although things might not always be perfect, that is okay. We all have different levels of success with various diet plans depending solely on our body's needs. It all depends on our body size, health issues, nutrient deficiencies, food intolerance's, activity level, age and genetics.  If you want to drop the lbs. then, you must estimate how much you personally should eat per day to lose that weight. Then, apply that amount to the balanced diet that your body needs and watch pounds drop away.

 The Harris-Benedict equation helps you estimate your basal metabolic rate, or BMR, which is how many calories you need daily to maintain your weight independent of daily activity and exercise. Many online calculators use this equation to give you a quick answer, but you can put pencil to paper to figure it out on your own. Plug your numbers into the following: 655 + (4.35 x your weight in pounds) + (4.7 x your height in inches) – (4.7 x your age in years). For a 40-year old, 5-foot, 5-inch woman weighing 160 pounds, the result comes out to 1,468 calories, for example

Listen you your body and trust yourself.

Make sure you're consuming enough calories in your eating window.

Make sure you're getting adequate nutrition.

Make sure you're eating enough healthy fats from sources like pastured animals, extra virgin olive oil, avocado oil, grass fed butter and/or egg yolks (if you don't have a food intolerance), avocados, fatty fish, etc.

Embrace mindfulness, meditation, and have social support.

Pay attention to your overall stress levels. You don't want to stress out your adrenal glands.

Get enough rest, let go of resentment, forgive others and be happy.

Do not fast for longer than 24 hours at a time

✓ Ideally fast for 12 to 16 hours

✓ Do not fast on consecutive days during your first two to three weeks of fasting (for instance, if you do a 16-hour fast, do it three days a week instead of seven)

✓ Drink plenty of fluids (bone broth, herbal tea, water) during your fast

✓ only do light exercise on fasting days, such as yoga, walking, jogging, and gentle stretching

✓ You want to eat clean, nutrient dense foods that feed your body.

✓ Some people fast 4:3 or 5:2 which means they eat 4 or 5 days during the week and fast 2 or 3 non-consecutive days of the week.

Always listen to your body. And do what works best for you. Make sure you Visit your doctor and share your interest in IF.

## Keeping your blood sugar stable

Keeping your blood sugar stable throughout the day is important. You don't want your blood sugar to drop nor get to high. Eating breakfast does jump-start your digestion and fire up your metabolism, as well as helping the body regulate blood sugar levels. Also, when you skip breakfast it makes your adrenal glands respond by secreting a hormone called cortisol. Cortisol then tells the liver to produce more glucose, bringing blood sugar levels back to normal. What happens when you have too much cortisol? It collects around your midsection. Cortisol is that hormone that is involved in the "flight or fight" response. Before you go grab that donut or high carb breakfast remember the word, metabolic syndrome.

Metabolic syndrome is caused by chronic hyperglycemia (high blood sugar). When you gobble down too many carbs, the pancreas secretes insulin to move excess glucose from the blood into the cells where glucose is used to produce energy. But over time, the cells lose the ability to respond to insulin. After so long of your insulin knocking at your front door of the cells. The cells stop hearing them. The pancreas responds by pumping out even more insulin (knocking louder) in an effort to get glucose into the cells, and this eventually causes insulin resistance. So with all this being said how should you handle breakfast?

Although I intermittent fast 3 days out of the week, I still eat breakfast after a few hours of waking. Start off by drinking a full 16 oz. glass of freshly squeezed lemon water on an empty stomach. Warm lemon water serves as the perfect good morning drink, pick-me-up drink, as it aids the digestive system being a rich source of nutrients like calcium, potassium, vitamin C and pectin fiber, phosphorus and magnesium. It also plays the role of blood purifier; has great antistatic properties; helps reduce pain and inflammation in joints and knees as it dissolves uric acid, strengthens the liver by providing energy to the liver enzymes: helps replenish body salts especially after a hard sweaty workout session: helps with body hydration, constipation; reduces phlegm; freshens breath: gives your immune system a boost; reduces inflammation; can help relieve or prevent digest problems like bloating, intestinal gas, and heartburn; and lastly weight loss; Breakfast doesn't have to be what people traditionally call breakfast foods. A salad, cup of soup, a cup of broth, a smoothie or even left over from the dinner the night before.

Food isn't just fuel it also has a major impact on your life. The foods you consume is information that is being sent to throughout your body and it will adjust accordingly to what is its being fed. Your GI tract doesn't just digest and absorb food. You see the GI tract has its own little powerful city among itself. This independently working nervous system (aka the enteric nervous system) has neurotransmitters, hormones, chemical messengers, enzymes, and bacteria along with being the home to 70 percent of your body's entire immune system! The quality of food does matter. Your GI tract also is the boss of your metabolism which it tells your metabolism to burn or store body fat based on the quality of calories. When a person is constantly feeding their body a food that they have an allergy or sensitivity to this creates a constant inflammatory response that will disrupt your life in many ways. Listening to your body is a great way to see if your body is having reactions to food sensitivities or an allergy. This is a list of things that can be associated with having a food allergy.

Chronic pain

Arthritis

Asthma

Nutrient deficiencies

Mood disorders

Skin conditions

Autoimmune disorders

Cognitive disorders

Learning disabilities

Insomnia

Weight gain

Migraines

Kidney and gallbladder problems

ADD/ADHD

Narcolepsy

Addiction

Kidney problems


One thing we have learned is each of us are unique and have our very own biochemistry that sets us apart from everyone else. Although we might share the same common traits and perhaps the same overlapping metabolic tendencies. We can't continue to say that one-size-fits-all when it comes to our very own unique body chemistry. There are over 7 billion people on this planet and we come in all different shapes, colors and sizes. With this being said wouldn't you think the one-size-fits-all- approach to losing weight wouldn't work since we are we are all unique.

Your body adapts to what your feeding it, the nutrients that are supplied are being processed differently and are sent to where its need. Just like a car, each item has its own function and you can run a car efficiently without every part working as it should.  The proteins, fats, and carbs are all converted into fuel using many different metabolic processes.

This is a short term trial. This list of foods below can be disrupting your life and you are just unaware. Keeping a food journal will allow you to be able to keep track of how these foods affect your body once you start to reintroduce them after a 3-week grace period from them.

# The Health Benefits of Fermented Foods

There are incredible health benefits when you start incorporating fermented foods to your diet. Fermented foods can help rebalance the gut flora and assist in the recovery from gut imbalances like Candida yeast overgrowth. However, every fermented food isn't created the same and is made different. Reading labels will help you determine what has and hasn't been added to it. This will let you know if it's safe for you to eat. Some additives are used the speed up the real fermentation process. Companies have been known to add sugars, preservatives, colorings, sodium benzoate or cheap vinegars. Did you know that many yogurts by the time they reach the store shelves contain no probiotic bacteria at all? Start reading the labels, you want to purchase fermented foods but try to find ones with organic ingredients, no sugars added, made with salt not vinegar and unpasteurized. Why you ask?  Fermented foods naturally have residual sweetness from the natural sugars in the food, so there is no need for these added sugars and let's not forget that Candida feeds on sugar. Also, we are trying to eliminate the un-necessary consumption of extra pesticides and chemicals therefore purchasing organic should be a no brainer. Lastly, pasteurization and sterilization kill the beneficial bacteria. Remember the enzymes in the food are destroyed by pasteurizing. Those enzymes help you to digest foods more easily and are needed to help you digest food more easily.

*A great resource on the topic is The Art of Fermentation by Sandor Katz.*

Did you know that your gut is the largest component of your immune system? It introduces friendly bacteria into your digestive system that helps to keep illness's at bay and they are rich in live bacteria that help us absorb nutrients along with maintain proper microbiome gut balance. Research has proven that gut health could affect inflammation, allergies and autoimmune disorders in the body as a whole. Around 1,000 different species of bugs live in your gut. We acquire them at birth (initially in the birth canal) and during the early years of childhood.

Your gut has been linked to contributing to weight loss and for overall improvement of numerous symptoms, including depression, anxiety, brain fog, skin problems, hormonal issues, immune weaknesses, digestive problems, and fatigue.

A healthy microbiome can transform our endocrine, immune, digestive, and nervous systems. So why not start eating fermented foods and give that microbiome some support? Maybe I am jumping the gun but I'd like to call fermented foods part of the new generation of Super foods.

More often than none many people suffer from an imbalance in the gut flora. There are more pathogenic bacteria in the gut then there are beneficial bacteria. An imbalance in the gut flora can contribute to leaky gut (intestinal permeability) which is one of the requirements for developing an autoimmune disease (such as Hashimoto's) as per Dr. Alessio Fassano who is one of the lead researchers on leaky gut disorders.

Dr. Alessio Fassano goes on to say," Rebalancing the gut bacteria will lead to normalization of leaky gut and therefore help to manage autoimmune conditions. Rebalancing can be done through diet (fermented foods), probiotics, digestive enzymes and/or medications."

Our beneficial bacteria are affected by processed foods, sugar intake, antibiotics, acid-reducing medications, toxins, and chronic stress.

# Not all fermented foods are Created Equal

You should avoid all types of unfermented soy products. All soy foods are high in copper. Copper also suppresses the thyroid and usually when someone is suffering from a fungal infection, they will also be suffering from a low thyroid condition called hypothyroidism.

Proper fermentation must be done with salt, NOT vinegar. Salt is antimicrobial in nature, and will inhibit the growth of putrefying bacteria while the lactic acid preserves the vegetables. Also, salt aids in the proper activation of enzymes. The salt should preferably be non-iodized and unprocessed as this contains minerals that help the lactobacilli grow.

Most fermented foods you can buy in supermarket jars or cans have been pasteurized and cooked at high heat, killing any friendly bacteria. High levels of sodium are the downside to savory fermented foods such as pickles, sauerkraut, kimchi, miso and soy sauce. Opt for low-sodium products when possible, or make your own to control added salt; in any case, use in moderation. We need to get those friendly bacteria – and not too much unfriendly sugars and sodium.

Great fermented food options that can be certified organic include:

Sauerkraut

Kimchi

Yogurt (Not dairy, use coconut yogurt)

Kefir

Kombucha (be careful with this, as the sugar content can be too high in some cases)

Pickles

Here is a brief history of fermentation from the Weston Price Foundation website:

It may seem strange to us that, in earlier times, people knew how to preserve vegetables for long periods without the use of freezers or canning machines through the process of lacto-fermentation. Lactic acid is a natural preservative that inhibits putrefying bacteria. Starches and sugars in vegetables and fruits are converted into lactic acid by the many species of lactic-acid-producing bacteria...The ancient Greeks understood that important chemical changes took place during this type of fermentation. Their name for this change was "alchemy." Like the fermentation of dairy products, preservation of vegetables and fruits by the process of lacto-fermentation has numerous advantages beyond those of simple preservation. The proliferation of lactobacilli in fermented vegetables enhances their digestibility and increases vitamin levels. These beneficial organisms produce numerous helpful enzymes as well as antibiotic and anticarcinogenic substances. Their main by-product, lactic acid, not only keeps vegetables and fruits in a state of perfect preservation but also promotes the growth of healthy flora throughout the intestine.

Health Benefits of Probiotics:

Relief of stress and anxiety

Reduces digestive discomfort

Improves mood gut-brain signaling

Protects against free radicals

Anti-inflammatory properties

Improves digestive health

Allergy prevention

Cholesterol reduction

Improves liver health

Natural Probiotics

There are different types of probiotics. Some are pills, powders, or capsules that contain billions of live bacteria and will help to replenish your microbiome. Fermented foods are more of a nature type of probiotic. They carry live bacteria plus many other crucial nutrients. Many cultures all around the world has their own recipes for fermented foods.

## Kombucha for your Armpits!!!

Aluminum-based antiperspirants may increase the risk for breast cancer, Alzheimer's disease and kidney disease. (Scientists noticed that dialysis patients who had these high aluminum levels were more likely to develop dementia too.) Our bodies are supposed to sweat. Sweat isn't inherently stinky either. In fact, it's nearly odorless. The stench comes from bacteria that break down from one of two types of sweat on your skin. Deodorant advertisers have done a pretty neat job of convincing us that we're disgustingly smelly people who in fact need to be refined and save our stinky selves by their products. We've been wonderfully brainwashed into thinking sweating is a bad thing. Sweating from the heat, sweating from exercise, and sweating from stress are all different, chemically speaking. Stress sweat smells the worst. That's because smelly sweat is only produced by one of the two types of sweat glands called the apocrine glands, which are usually in areas with lots of hair—like our armpits, the groin area, and scalp. The odor is the result of the bacteria that break down the sweat once it's released onto your skin.

*Fun fact: While women have more sweat glands than men, men's sweat glands produce more sweat.*

No one can force you to become more aware of what you put on your body and what you put in your body. What you eat is just as important as what you put on your body. Adjusting your life, reading labels and catering to your specific health needs isn't easy but it will benefit you in the long run. This is one of the smartest decisions that you can make. Not only will you start to look and feel better but think of the medical cost that you could be saving your future self.

Did you know that it takes 26 seconds for the chemicals in personal body care products to enter into your bloodstream?

Endocrine disruptors are tricky chemicals that play on our bodies. They increase production of certain hormones; decreasing production of others; imitating hormones; turning one hormone into another; interfering with hormone signaling; telling cells to die prematurely; competing with essential nutrients; binding to essential hormones; accumulating in organs that produce hormones. You can start avoiding these chemicals by starting with detoxifying your beauty routine.

Let's talk about our under arms. I stopped using commercial deodorant quickly when I discovered all the harmful ingredients it has in it and quite frankly aluminum chlorohdrate or aluminum zirconium found in commercial brands wasn't something extra that I cared to willingly put on my skin. On my underarms no doubt where it's so close to my breasts.

Frankly, it took several weeks for my body to get use to the non-use of chemical loaded store bought deodorants. I didn't enjoy feeling like I was plagued with BO for those weeks until my body became adjusted. If you've tried homemade deodorants and they didn't work at all covering up those stinky under arm pits of yours. The odor is the result of the bacteria colonizing you're in armpits. Have you ever thought about adding more bacteria?

## Why not Kombucha for your armpits?

1 tbsp. cocoa butter

-1 tbsp. coconut oil

-1 tbsp. shea butter

-1 tbsp. beeswax

-2 1/2 tbsp. arrowroot powder

-1 tbsp. baking soda

-1/4 tsp. vitamin E oil

-10 drops essential oil of your choice

-2 capsules powdered probiotics


I like lavender or grapefruit or any citrus scent. Men can use cypress/bergamot

Small Mason jar with lid

This is a small recipe you can double our triple it if you'd like.

Mix baking soda and arrowroot together. Melt your coconut oil, shea butter, and cocoa butter in 1 minute's intervals in the microwave in a microwave-safe bowl. Stir during each interval. Mix all ingredients (the baking soda and arrowroot powder) with the oil. Pour into clean small Mason jar. Add your essential oil and vitamin E to the Mason jar; close with the lid. Give it a good shake to combine the essential oil with the other mixture. Allow it to cool for about 30 minutes or the consistency of pudding, open capsules of probiotics and add powder to mixture. Stir with spatula quickly to combine. Allow to completely cool. It usually takes overnight.  I use my finger to scoop out what I need to rub on my underarms.

Why you need to get rid of soy gluten/grains, Legumes, lectins, peanuts, nightshades, Dairy, caffeine, corn, eggs, sugar + artificial sweeteners.... Until you know if you have a food intolerance to these items.

Things you eat can interfere with your body's ability to heal itself.

## Avoid SOY!!!!

Soy not only disrupts hormones by mimicking estrogen in your body but it also causes inflammation, contributes to leaky gut syndrome and most likely has been genetically modified (GMO). Start reading your labels. You will be surprised how companies will sneak in soy.

Brilliant marketing campaigns have lead you to believe that soy products are healthy but in fact it's completely the opposite. Soy products are not healthy foods. Eating soy frequently can potentially lead to numerous other health issues.

For centuries, Asian people have been consuming fermented soy products such as natto, tempeh, and soy sauce, and enjoying the health benefits. Fermented soy does not wreak havoc on your body like unfermented soy products do.

The issue with soy is most soy today contains something called phytoestrogens, and these phytoestrogens are estrogen mimickers in the body. And so, if you're a male consuming extra estrogen, it's going to give you more feminine characteristics.

If you're a woman consuming foods that increase estrogen levels, it's going to increase your risk of breast cancer, cervical cancer, PCOS (polycystic ovary syndrome) and other hormone imbalance-related disorders.

Many have felt as if they needed a diary substitute since they couldn't tolerate dairy. Actually your body was doing you an even bigger favor.

For starters, some chemicals such as isoflavones, found in soy products like soy milk or edamame, can intercept your thyroid's ability to make hormones if you're not getting enough iodine.

Soybeans are one of the crops that are being genetically modified. Since 1997 GMO soybeans are being used in an increasing number of products.

Dr. Kaayla Daniel, author of The Whole Soy Story, points out thousands of studies linking soy to malnutrition, digestive distress, immune-system breakdown, thyroid dysfunction, cognitive decline, reproductive disorders and infertility—even cancer and heart disease. Here is just a sampling of the health effects that have been linked to soy consumption:

Breast cancer

Brain damage

Infant abnormalities

Thyroid disorders

Kidney stones

Immune system impairment

Severe, potentially fatal food allergies

Impaired fertility

Danger during pregnancy and nursing


Final thoughts on Soy: Soy is terrible – contains trypsin inhibitors, is a source of xenoestrogens, even if it's organic, and if it's GMO, it also comes with a lot of glyphosate and other pesticide residues. Avoid it like the black plague....

# Avoid caffeine!!

Caffeine adds stress to your adrenal glands and the endocrine system. Caffeine will stimulate you adrenals causing them to adrenaline and cortisol in the exact same way as they do during a 'fight or flight' reaction. Caffeine gives you a false boost in energy before the fall to fatigue.

Your thyroid is very sensitive to stimulants. It only confuses your already overworked system.

If you must have coffee, try to limit it to one cup of coffee a day.

As for caffeinated soda, this beverage is a loaded with empty calories, a crazy amount of sugar and then top if off with the caffeine. You can purchase soda water without sodium and squeeze a lemon or lime into it.

## Avoid dairy and gluten

Most people don't realize that they have a very common food allergies to gluten and dairy. A1 casein is a protein found in cow's milk. The A1 casein and gluten both can cause Leaky Gut Syndrome. This will increase inflammation and tax your already low hormone producing thyroid gland.  When you have a "Leaky gut" it allows particles to leak from your digestive tract and travel freely through your bloodstream. This puts your immune system on high alert to neutralize all of these threats. After a while of the constant abuse from your leaky gut and eventually puts your body in a state of chronic inflammation and next setting you on the path to develop an autoimmune disease where your immune system becomes so stressed and confused that it begins attacking your own tissue by mistake. So the next time you go to eat that cheeseburger keep in mind that since you have a leaky gut that was originally caused by gluten and dairy consumption, your willingly allowing their proteins to  travel freely into your bloodstream, where they trigger an attack from your immune system.  I use ghee for cooking very frequently. The clarifying process also removes casein.  I also use coconut milk.  In my research, these are a safer way to eat dairy if you must any type of raw dairy – milk, butter, cheese, cream, sour cream, cream cheese, ice cream, heavy cream, yogurt and any type of pasteurized grass-fed dairy of cream, butter, and ghee.

Gluten intolerance is pretty common than previously recognized.  It's a major trigger for autoimmune conditions. By removing wheat, barley, and rye products, as well as corn, oats, millet, and coffee you are allowing yourself to heal.

## Avoid Nightshades

There have been really ZERO scientific articles written or studied about nightshade sensitivity, chronic pain, or arthritis. However, you can do a search on the internet and find many people who has been affected by nightshades. They seem to aggravate arthritis, fibromyalgia, or other chronic pain syndromes. I seem to be sensitive to nightshades; they cause me a variety of symptoms, like difficulty concentrating, pounding heart, muscle/nerve/joint pain, and ungodly-long nights of insomnia. Pay attention to your body, we all are different and are affected in different ways.  There is no harm in exploring other potential culprits if you are having pain, gastrointestinal issues, and neurological/psychiatric symptoms.

Not all plants are created equal and they have a way of defending themselves from plant predators like yourself. Some plants are a wonderful source of essential nutrients but if you think they have survived millions of years just to be picked, plucked and eaten? Oh boy have we ever been wrong! They are living and want to survive where they can pass on their genes to their next generation. Plants are fantastic at supplying our body with vitamins, minerals, antioxidants and other nutrients but not all plants are created equal. Sometimes plants can actually do more harm than good.

If you have an autoimmune disease, arthritis, gout, osteoporosis and ongoing inflammation eliminating nightshades can help you heal. Nightshades has Alkaloids, Calcitrol and high in lectins.  Lectins are plants as a natural pesticide.  It is a "sticky" molecules that tend to attach to the walls of the intestine and can exacerbate a leaky gut.  Calcitriol is a hormone that signals your body that you need more calcium in your blood.  Therefore your body starts to store calcium deposits in soft tissues, such as tendons and ligaments.

Last but not least Alkaloids which cause stress and inflammation in your body.

Nightshades include:

Potatoes (not sweet potatoes or yams)

Tomatoes

Eggplant

All peppers (not peppercorn), including hot peppers, chili peppers, sweet peppers and paprika

Ashwaganda

Gogi berries

Cape gooseberries (not normal gooseberries)

Ground cherries

# Avoid Sugar and Artificial sweeteners

Sugar is nothing but empty calories and is hidden in everything that we eat that is processed or pre-packaged by mankind. Sugar is addictive like most modern day drugs and it activates the same brain system as drugs such as nicotine and cocaine. It is responsible for a large number of health conditions that plague humans in the 21st century. The king of artificial sweeteners was allowed to the market in 1981 when the U.S. Commissioner of Food and Drugs, Arthur Hull Hayes, overruled FDA panel suggestions, as well as consumer concerns. Aspartame is a neurotoxin that interacts with natural organisms, as well as synthetic medications, producing a wide range of proven disorders and syndromes. Artificial sweeteners has been linked to weight gain, decreased vision, severe PMS, phobia's, hyperactivity in children, chronic fatigue syndrome, fibromyalgia, birth defects headaches and migraine's.

# Avoid Legumes, Lectin and peanuts.

Scientists discovered lectins 1884 while on their quest while investigating different blood types. They also found that lectins cause an inflammatory reaction in the body. Lectins are proteins that bind to carbohydrates or glycoproteins and they allow cells to bind or communicate with each other. Scientists believe that lectins are part of a plant's protection system.

Fun facts: Did you know that 94% of humans are born with antibodies to the lectins in peanuts?

Legumes contain lectins. Peanuts are a legume and it also carries aflatoxins which is a type of mold.

Did you know that lectins can simulate weight gain?

List of legumes

Alfalfa

Asparagus bean

Asparagus pea

Baby lima bean

Black bean

Black-eyed pea

Black turtle bean

Boston bean

Boston navy bean

Broad bean

Cannellini bean

Chickpeas

Chili bean

Cranberry bean

Dwarf bean

Egyptian bean

Egyptian white broad bean

English bean

Fava bean

Fava coceira

Field pea

French green bean

Frijol bola roja

Frijole negro

Great northern bean

Green bean

Green and yellow peas

Kidney bean

Lentils

Lespedeza

Licorice

Lima bean

Madagascar bean

Mexican black bean

Mexican red bean

Molasses face bean

Mung bean

Mung pea

Mungo bean

Navy bean

Pea bean

Peanut

Peruvian bean

Pinto bean

Red bean

Red clover

Red eye bean

Red kidney bean

Rice bean

Runner bean

Scarlet runner bean

Small red bean

Snow pea

Southern pea

Sugar snap pea

Soybean

Wax bean

White vlover

White kidney bean

White pea bean


## *Avoid Corn*

I bet you didn't know that corn is an actually a grain that is full of Omega 6s that produce hormones that support inflammation. It is genetically modified food and continues to be re-engineered in more ways that we can imagine. Although corn doesn't have gluten in it, it can still aggravate auto immune disorders. Corn contains lectins and we can't digest it. Not to mention it's loaded with pesticides.

# Fighting Constipation, electrolyte imbalance, leg cramps and avoiding the Keto flu

## Fighting Constipation on Keto AIP

Bowel movements is your body's way to get rid of waste buildup. Don't worry sometimes people do tend to find themselves constipated. You've changed the way you're eating and for some it might be harder for their body to digest or adjust to this new way of eating. Also, when you are in ketosis, your body loses more water as it burns up the carb stores and makes ketones therefore your body might not be getting get enough fluid, so your colon will pull extra from your stools and this will can certainly slow things down in your gut and cause constipation.

We have two types of poopers in this world: Type A has their pooping down to a science. They go every day at the same time and usually (if they can help it) in the same toilet. (This is me)  Then there's Type B. This group doesn't go that often and has no real ritual to its toilet habits.  So, you may ask, is one healthier than the other? The answer is no. Everyone is different. There really is no "normal" habit for pooping.  The average person poops approximately once a day—about 1 ounce of stool for each 12 pounds of her or his body weight. That means a person weighing 160 pounds produces an average of just under a pound of poop each day. Poop is made up of 75% water the remaining parts are made from a mixture of dead bacteria that helped us to digest our food, living bacteria, protein, indigestible fiber, and waste materials from the liver and intestines. Don't start to worry if you bathroom habits change. It's going to happen. We go on vacation & things happen in our lives. As long as your bathroom trips don't cause pain or discomfort you are pretty much okay. Your digestive system works all day and every day, so it's okay if you experience changes from time to time.  If you have constipation or diarrhea that lasts for longer than weeks at a time or blood in your stool you need to

Check with your doctor.

Here are a few things you can do to help if you experience constipation.

Eat More Fermented foods- like sauerkraut, kimchi, and pickles for probiotic bacteria and prebiotic fiber

Drink more health fats- like olives, avocados

Drink More Water

Consume More MCT Oil-MCT (medium chain triglycerides) oil has a natural laxative effect you won't find in other types of oil

Add Himalayan Sea Salt to your Water-Salt water can counteract constipation. Add a small dash of salt into a glass of water twice a day. Try this mixture an hour or so before eating on an empty stomach.

Important: If you have high blood pressure, don't try this. You already know you are limited to 1500 milligrams (mgs) of sodium per day.

Add extra blueberries-

Add an extra avocado

Add 1 teaspoon of organic honey

Make sure your eating plenty of low GI vegetables

Add a daily probiotic, prebiotic and digestive enzyme

Add a fermented fish oil supplement

Drink an extra cup of green tea it's a natural diuretic

Get out and exercise

Add 1 tablespoon of coconut oil to your warm water

Make sure your taking a high quality mulit-vitamin-I use Garden of life

## What are Electrolytes?

There are 4 basic electrolyte minerals potassium, magnesium, calcium and sodium. If one or more of these are off balance you can experience the Keto flu, leg cramps, or an electrolyte imbalance. You may find that you are going to the bathroom more than usual. The body begins to get rid of more water because the reduction in carbs tells your kidneys to release more stored sodium and you're not eating crap anymore that has all that added extra sodium. You should always try to aim to drink have your body weight in water. It's easy to figure it out by taking your body weight and divide it by two. Say you say 150 lbs. that means you will need to drink a minimum of 75. Ounces. So, it's very important that you stay hydrated along with electrolytes so you won't experience flu. I have done shots of pickle juice, drank extra broths that had Himalayan sea salt in it, ate foods higher in potassium like spinach and avocado, ate foods higher in magnesium like spinach, avocado and fatty fish.

Electrolytes are specific nutrients in our bodies crucial for important functions like:

Muscle contractions

Heartbeat regulation

Body temperature control

Bladder control

Energy production

Neurological functions

Here are a few things you can do to help if you think you have an electrolyte imbalance.

Add 1-2 bouillon cubes to water-

Drink an extra cup of bone, vegetable or fish broth

Add more potassium-rich foods, such as broccoli, avocado, salmon and chicken breast

If you are experiencing leg cramps your magnesium can be low-

You can add Magnesium glycinate or Magnesium malate- make sure you follow directions


## *Homemade Keto Electrolyte Drink #1*

Aloe Vera juice has been used for thousands of years and for fantastic reasons. Aloe contains vitamins A, B12, C, and E, creating a powerful antioxidant effect. Natural enzymes which reduce inflammation and help break down sugars and fats.  Minerals like calcium, chromium, copper, selenium, magnesium, manganese, potassium, sodium, and zinc. Four plant steroids which are fatty acids and have anti-inflammatory along with antiseptic, properties. Last but not least Aloe contains 20 different amino acids, including seven of the eight essential amino acids. Himalayan sea salt has over 84 minerals and trace elements, including calcium, magnesium, potassium, copper and iron. This sea salt comes from one of the oldest and richest salt fields in the world. It is located near Punjab region of Pakistan about 190 miles from the Himalayas. Many believe it is the dried remnants of the original, primal sea. Never use table salt because it is 97.5 percent to 99.9 percent sodium chloride, highly processed and has no remaining minerals. Most table salts have added iodine where Himalayan sea salt has natural iodine and table salts have an added anti-clumping agent called yellow prussiate of soda which is a health-hazardous. Lemons have calcium, potassium, magnesium and natural sodium. Ginger contains potassium.

***Caution: Aloe Vera can interact with certain medications and aggravate a few conditions like kidney disease. Always check with your health care provider before starting a new regime. ***


1/3 teaspoon Himalayan sea salt

2 oz. unsweetened pure aloe Vera juice

1 teaspoon fresh lemon juice

24oz. filter water

Mix and drink.


## Homemade Keto Electrolyte Drink #2

I prefer to juice this but you can put it in a blender too. The main star here is celery. Celery helps heal the gut,  calcium, silicon, vitamins K, A, B1, B2, B6 and C, minerals potassium, folic acid, calcium, magnesium, iron, phosphorus, sodium, reduces blood pressure, helps to purify the bloodstream, balancing the body's pH level, helps to neutralize any acidity in the body, replaces lost electrolytes, re-hydrates the body, natural laxative effect and its Anti-Inflammatory. Cucumbers are high in potassium. Spinach, kale, collards, and mustard greens have a nice amount of magnesium, potassium, and calcium. Lemons have calcium, potassium, magnesium and natural sodium. Ginger contains potassium.

What's the difference between juicing and blending you ask? Juicing discards the indigestible fiber. Without this fiber, your digestive system doesn't have to work as hard to break down the food to absorb the nutrients. Blending helps to create a slow more even release of nutrients into the blood stream and avoids blood sugar spikes. I find that smoothies are more filling and less expensive than juicing but I do love to juice.

6 stalks of celery

½ peeled lemon

Small bunch of parsley

¼ inch piece of peeled ginger

1/2 cucumber

1 cup of Spinach, kale, collards, or mustard greens (your preference)

*** (If you have hypothyroidism replace Spinach, kale, collards, or mustard greens with 1 cup of romaine lettuce.) ****

16 oz. of water (if you're blending and not juicing)...

# Incase I've missed some vital information here is 33 other Tips along with a recap of some pretty important stuff to help you begin to heal

This is certainly a life-changing experience. Once you decide to become healthier you will find that you will become a whole new person. Keep in mind before anything changes in your life you have to open yourself to the possibilities of change. This is the first step in the journey of gaining knowledge. Personal growth, an open mind and the possibility for change. I've written many truths in this book and I hope many can be applied to your life. Please allow this wisdom to be communicated within you. You can find all the references and resources in the back of the book.

How would you define good health? Logically one would define good health as absence of a disease or following some sort of ground rules that avoid developing a disease. i certainly hope this book has helped you gain knowledge to start guiding you in the redevelopment and healing of your body. I hoped you have begun to understand how to fix your gut, strengthen your immunity and fight inflammation with an autoimmune approach. By removing things from your life you can stop autoimmune reactions in the body. Along with helping to reset those adrenals, boosting that energy and doing a little ass kicking to those hormones that have decided to act like a wild college student and pull an all-nighter the day before final exams.

Most of us don't realize until we've been diagnosed with a chronic disease or start experiencing symptoms that every single function in our body depends upon the food we eat, the water and the chemicals that we allow to come in contact with our bodies on a daily basis.

Your health doesn't have to be a difficult situation but a positive realization that things need to change.

I wrote this book because, just like you, I've suffered from inflammation, autoimmunity, a leaky gut and a sluggish immune system.

No matter the resistance that you get, stay true to yourself and your purpose.

What you discover in my book can be the key to your peace of mind and a healthier, happier you.

The full true benefit of the KETO AIP is seen when you take the whole system into account.

# BE YOUR OWN HEALTH ADVOCATE

Research and study. No one needs you more than yourself. After being diagnosed my priorities were made clearer. I had to start listening to my body, stop taking my health for granted and continuing to research to figure out what I needed to do to "fix me".

A lack of knowledge is a lack of power....

## 1. Look into getting a Knowledgeable Health Practitioner:

The very first thing that you need to do is look into getting a knowledgeable holistic health practitioner!

There are six principals of neuropath medicine:

1. Do no Harm
2. Allow the healing power of nature
3. Find the cause
4. The doctor is a teacher not a drug pusher
5. Prevention
6. Treat the whole person not the symptoms

The main reason why you should work with a knowledgeable health practitioner is its patient-centered medical healing at its best. Unfortunately, when it comes to your body there isn't a one size fits all approach to dealing with it and often times you are left still searching for the answers to your symptoms when all you want is your zest for life back. A knowledgeable health practitioner will care for you as an individual as they won't look at your body as a whole they will treat each individual body symptom, imbalance and dysfunction. They will take into consideration the whole person, including physical, mental and spiritual aspects, when treating a health condition or promoting wellness. I want you to understand that you are made up of interdependent parts and if one part is not working properly, all the other parts will be affected. A knowledgeable health practitioner certainly moves from the confusion of the "one size fits all treatment" approach that we know isn't working to the one that will cater to what your body needs. Let's not forget that each of us are a unique case and unless you get a proper thorough clinical evaluation, trying to figure what medical advise you need online is dubious at best.

## 2. Start making your underarm deodorant

Deodorant and antiperspirants impair the underarm lymph nodes. Aluminum-based compounds are the active ingredients in antiperspirants. Sweating is a necessity in life. There are roughly three million sweat glands pumping out as much as 14 liters/ 3 gallons of water a day. Sweat, as stinky and uncomfortable as it can be at times, is a natural and healthy part of life, helping to cool the body, release toxins and helps to maintain normal body temperatures. Sweat isn't inherently stinky either. In fact, it's nearly odorless. The stench comes from bacteria that break down from one of two types of sweat on your skin. Deodorant advertisers have done a pretty neat job of convincing us that we're disgustingly smelly people who in fact need to be refined and save our stinky selves by their products. We've been wonderfully brainwashed into thinking sweating is a bad thing. Sweating from the heat, sweating from exercise, and sweating from stress are all different, chemically speaking. Stress sweat smells the worst. That's because smelly sweat Is only produced by one of the two types of sweat glands called the Apocrine glands, which are usually in areas with lots of hair—like our Armpits, the groin area, and scalp. The odor is the result of the bacteria that break down the sweat once it's released onto your skin.

Important Note: Aluminum fluoride is the compound often found in the brains of Alzheimer's patients. Aluminum can be found in cheaply made pots and pans, antacids, vaccines, flu shots, tap water, baking powder, deodorants and antiperspirants, and most food imported from China.  Causes Alzheimer's, Parkinson's and other dementia disorders.

Deodorant Recipe

Ingredients

1/2 c. baking soda

1/2 c. arrowroot powder or ½ cup of cornstarch

5 tbsp. unrefined virgin coconut oil

10 drops of grapefruit essential oil or lavender essential oil

You can pick your favorite scent. I like lavender or grapefruit.


Empty deodorant stick or Mason jar

Directions

Mix baking soda and arrowroot together.

Melt your coconut oil in the microwave in a microwave safe bowl.

Mix all ingredients the baking soda and arrowroot powder with the oil, pour into clean small Mason jar, (or your empty stick container) add your essential oil to the Mason jar or the empty stick container, using a wooden Popsicle stick, give it a good stir to mix everything. Close you're the lid. Once you mix that essential oil in the bowl, it can only be used for the purpose of making your deodorant. Everything you've used is edible except the essential oils.

This will take roughly 24 hours to set. It will thicken up. I use my finger to scrape what I need out of the Mason jar and scoop it across my underarm. This will last you for a good 6 months!


Natural Tooth Paste Recipe

Natural Peppermint Toothpaste

1/2 cup coconut oil

3 Tablespoons of baking soda

15 drops of peppermint food grade essential oil

Melt to soften the coconut oil. Mix in other ingredients and stir well. Place your mixture into small glass jar. Allow it to cool completely. When ready to use just dip toothbrush in and scrape small amount onto bristles.

Homemade Coconut Oil Toothpaste Recipe

6 tbsp. coconut oil

6 tbsp. baking soda

15-20 drops of a food grade essential oil optional

Melt to soften the coconut oil. Mix in other ingredients and stir well. Place your mixture into small glass jar. Allow it to cool completely. When ready to use just dip toothbrush in and scrape small amount onto bristles.

## 3. Address Food sensitivities

If you allergic to certain foods it is will involve you're the immune system. You know that your immune system controls how your body defends itself. Your body see's inflammatory foods as invaders and will kick in your autoimmunity responses. For example if you have a food allergy to cow's milk, your immune system will see cow's milk as an invader. In-return your immune system overreacts by producing antibodies called Immunoglobulin E (IgE). These antibodies travel to cells that release chemicals, causing an allergic reaction to start fighting for your body. Being tested for food allergies or remove them from your diet for a couple of weeks or so to see if you feel better seems to be one of the easiest tasks to do.

## 4. Try OIL PULLING

An ancient Ayurvedic ritual dating back over 3,000 years, oil pulling involves placing a tablespoon of extra virgin organic cold pressed oil (I use coconut oil) into your mouth and then swishing it around for up to 20 minutes, minimum 5 minutes (pulling it between your teeth), before spitting it out.

Whatever you do, do not swallow the oil as you will ingest the toxins you are trying to wipe out. Afterwards requires brushing your teeth with an all-natural fluoride-free toothpaste, and rinsing your mouth out. And you're done! It really is that easy.

WHY OIL PULLING?

Oil pulling can really transform your health. Your mouth is the home to millions of bacteria, fungi, viruses and other toxins, the oil acts like a cleanser, pulling out the nasties before they get a chance to spread throughout the body.

This frees up the immune system, reduces stress, curtails internal inflammation and aids well-being.

This frees up the immune system, reduces stress, curtails internal inflammation and aids well-being.

## 5. Address nutritional deficiencies

Having nutritional deficiencies certainly adds gas to the fire. When you are deficient it can aggravate the symptoms: vitamin D, iron, omega-3 fatty acids, selenium, zinc, copper, vitamin A, the B vitamins, and iodine.

## 6. Address Chronic Candida

Did you know that an overload of Candida was picked up at birth or shortly thereafter? We were supposed to be getting good friendly bacteria from our mother's at birth, but "our" mother's had Candida overgrowth and unknowing passed it on to us. And over the years, our bodies has become more and more compromised. Your gut microbes could be dramatically affecting your thyroid health. There is a lot of misinformation and misunderstanding about Candida. Both from the medical profession and on the internet. It is easy to get fooled into thinking, as many sites will try to convince you, that all anyone needs to do is to take their product or buy their e-book. Of course, they will all have testimonies. What they don't tell you in those testimonies is how the Candida came back — in a month or two or in six months. However long it took for the Candida to overgrow enough to start causing symptoms again. It is important to know that dealing with Candida is not an easy fix.

## 7. Address Hormonal imbalances

Why it is that one person can eat all they want and never gain an inch, while someone else gains weight just looking at food? The fact is some people are wired to simply burn fat better than others. There are sneaky little things in your body that can halt your weight loss success. This is why you really need a Knowledgeable Board Certified Health Practitioner.

## 8. Address Magnesium deficiencies-

 Magnesium is necessary for metabolizing estrogen in the liver. Magnesium is a mineral that plays an important part in our health and well-being. It's one of the forgotten minerals and it's vital for many processes within the body. Magnesium helps to keep the nervous system healthy and to calm your nerves when you are stressed. In fact, did you know that magnesium is the first mineral depleted when you are stressed? So if you have any type of stress in your life magnesium is the first mineral that goes out the window. Magnesium is also an important mineral co-factor for enzymes that have biochemical reactions in the body. In other words, it plays a large role in digestive system health as it helps enzymes do their job as well as to loosen the body to relax and ease to support the metabolic processes.

Calming Magnesium Body Butter

1/2 cup cocoa butter

1/2 cup of coconut oil and melt

1/4 cup magnesium oil

Add 10 drops of lavender essential oil,

Add 10 drops cedarwood essential oil

Add 10 drops frankincense essential oil

Place a heat-safe glass measuring cup/bowl inside a pot that has 1-2 inches of simmering water over medium heat. Add the cocoa butter & Melt it in your double boiler until it's completely melted.


Remove the cocoa butter from heat, and add 1/2 cup extra virgin coconut oil to the melted cocoa butter and stir until completely the coconut oil has melted. Next add 1/4 cup magnesium oil to the mixture and combine. Place the mixture in the refrigerator to cool for about 30-60 minutes (until it is cooled completely). After the mixture has completely cooled and became a solid. Use a hand mixer or stand mixer to whip it. Start on low and increase speed slowly. Whip for about 3-5 minutes. Next add the 10 drops each of lavender essential oil, the 10 drops of cedar wood essential oil, and the 10 drops of frankincense essential oil. Scrape down the sides of the bowl and continue whipping for another 5 minutes or so, until the magnesium body butter is light and fluffy. The color of the magnesium body butter will change from yellow to a pale ivory and almost white color. Lastly put the magnesium body butter into mason jars and seal tightly with a lid. Make sure to label and date the top of the lid. This recipe makes enough for two 4 oz. glass jars.

## 9. Address the toxic burden

Did you know that it takes 26 seconds for the chemicals in personal body care products to enter into your bloodstream?

Endocrine disruptors are tricky chemicals that play on our bodies. They increase production of certain hormones; decreasing production of others; imitating hormones; turning one hormone into another; interfering with hormone signaling; telling cells to die prematurely; competing with essential nutrients; binding to essential hormones; accumulating in organs that produce hormones. One-way you can start avoiding these chemicals is by starting with detoxifying your beauty routine.

These are commonly found in items like antibacterial soap, deodorant, lotions, and makeup. These things are poisonous. Your skin is the largest organ in the body. Whatever you put on your skin goes into your body. I can't preach this enough. If you can't eat it, then don't apply it to your skin. These are endocrine disruptions. I understand this might not be 100% doable but every little bit helps your body. Every day we are exposed to a huge number of chemical toxins without our own doing. It's in our water, the pollution in our air, the insecticides and herbicides that are is sprayed on our food and the chemicals that are spray on our lawns. You can stop using toxic chemicals and start making your own soap, deodorant, lotions, and makeup. i have so many recipes in my book Awareness has Magic or you can google recipes.

The real reality is we are damaging our DNA and we are changing our genetic makeup for future generations. There was a study a few years back that said the umbilical cord of an average American baby has over 200 known chemicals in it. Eighty percent of the common chemicals that are used daily in this country, we know almost nothing about. Our children are being born toxic and we have no idea if these toxins are already doing some sort of damage their brains, their immune system, their reproductive system, and any other developing organs. Are we unknowingly setting ourselves up for failure in the womb, even before birth?

Scientists and researchers are concerned that many of these chemicals may be carcinogenic or wreak havoc with our hormones, our body's regulating system.

Most products have a warning label that is typed in bold "Keep out of Reach of Children".  As consumers, we believe that if our children don't ingest these products they will not be harmed by them. This can be far from the truth. Think about other common methods of exposure are through the skin and our respiratory tract. WE are along with our children are often in contact with the chemical residues housecleaning products do leave behind, by crawling, lying and sitting on the freshly cleaned floor.

Scientists at Norway's University of Bergen tracked 6,000 people, with an average age of 34 at the time of enrollment in the study, who used the cleaning products over a period of two decades, according to the research published in the American Thoracic Society's American Journal of Respiratory and Critical Care Medicine.

These chemicals can chemicals bind together.

Exposure to phthalates has been associated with lower IQ levels.

These chemicals can also be found in the shampoos, conditioners, body sprays, hair sprays, perfumes, make up, cleaning supplies, colognes, soap and nail polish that we use.

The results follow a study by French scientists in September 2017 that found nurses who used disinfectants to clean surfaces at least once a week had a 24 percent to 32 percent increased risk of developing lung disease.

Pesticides, herbicides, GMOs in our food, fluoride and chlorine and trace pharmaceutical residue in the water supplies, methane, carbon monoxide and industrial pollutants in the air, and the toxic chemicals in our everyday household products.

No wonder our bodies are completely bombarded and overwhelmed with the constant exposed to toxic chemicals through the air that we breathe, the water we drink, the foods we eat, and the personal care products and cleaning products we use.

The Centers of Disease Control found traces of 212 different chemicals in a group of people that they studied over the course of five years, and that's only the chemicals they tested for! Your body is absorbing all these toxins.

Nobody knows the effects of all these chemicals has on our bodies and yet thousands of chemicals are in regular use daily. By you having a higher toxic burden it puts a strain on your body and puts you at greater risk of developing an autoimmune disease.

It's not enough to be aware of all the outdoor chemicals that we are exposed to everyday but inside our homes we can have more power and control. We have to be more aware about using chemical cleaners, paints, glues, body lotions, toothpastes, underarm deodorants, hair products and pesticides. Instead start to begin to use products that don't pollute our very own bodies. We must read labels, make our own products and do our own research. I can't stress this enough. We must take a stand for our health. Stop using commercial products that are laced with unknown and harmful body damaging products.

## 10. Address the Lymphatic System

The lymphatic system is your body's natural detox system that is connected as part of your immune system and it is a complex drainage or "sewer" system that consists of glands, lymph nodes, the spleen, thymus gland, and tonsils. Many of us never realize just how important your lymphatic system is nor the fact that it plays one of the largest roles in our bodies by cleansing nearly every bodily cell by removing toxins, metabolic waste and so more. It's also cleanses our cells by absorbing excess fluids, fats, and toxins from our tissues. This waste is pushed into our blood stream where it can eventually be filtered out by the liver and kidneys. Not only is your lymphatic system responsible for flushing out the waste material of the body but it is also responsible for distributing nutrients to each and every part of our body.

## 11. Address Parasites and Heavy Metals

   Heavy metals weaken our body's defense system against foreign invaders and make it convenient for them to set up house. American's are not being protected as we should from pollution. We don't have to go to a 3rd world country or even a foreign country be subjected to contaminated water which can led to illnesses.  The pollution in our air, water, food supply, cleaning products, body products, commercial weed killers and chem trails in our environment. It's really hard not to have some sort of health issues that come from a heavy metal over load on our bodies. Just imagine commercial meat production, can goods and prepackaged foods. Heavy metals make a very acid environment which is very harmful to your gut flora where parasites and candida love to flourish.  Candida and parasites actually do serve a purpose in your body they are to protect us from the potentially fatal complications of heavy metal poisoning. They feed on heavy metals and store them within biofilms- buffering us from heavy metal overload.

## 12. Address your Gut

Your gut is your portal to health. It houses 80 percent of your immune system, and without your gut being healthy it is practically impossible to have a healthy immune system.  A leaky gut have been linked to hormonal imbalances, autoimmune diseases such as rheumatoid arthritis and Hashimotos thyroiditis, diabetes, chronic fatigue, fibromyalgia, anxiety, depression, eczema and rosacea, and that is just to name a few. It is said that all disease begin in the gut. So you can understand why a properly working digestive system (your gut) is vital to your health. Contrary to what we use to believe. We now know that having a leaky gut is one of the main reasons, and probably the beginning stage, for developing an autoimmune disease. Having a leaky gut means that the tight junctions that usually hold the walls of your intestines together have become loose, allowing undigested food particles, microbes, toxins, and more to leave your gut and enter your bloodstream. This will cause your body to become full of inflammation, which in return will start to trigger an autoimmune condition and if you already have an autoimmune condition it will certainly make it worse. Luckily for you. Your gut is made up of wonderful cells that can turn over very quickly, so you can start to heal your gut in as little as thirty days. Also things that you need to be aware of when addressing your gut is the over use of antibiotics, NSAIDS, and Stomach acid blockers.  Antibiotics are certainly one of the greatest advances in modern medicine when it was discovered in the 1940's. There are two types of germs that make people sick.  Bacteria and viruses. Antibiotics do not work against viruses and your body's own immune if given the chance can beat these little things.  Antibiotics are needed if you have a Bacterial infection. They cause illness by invading your body, multiplying, and interfering with normal bodily processes. Make sure you u know the difference of your illness before you are so quit to take that prescription of antibiotic.  You see, antibiotics doesn't know the difference between good or bad bacteria therefore it kills both.  There are some 20 traditional nonsteroidal anti-inflammatory drugs or NSAIDs, including aspirin, ibuprofen (Advil and Motrin), naproxen (Aleve), indomethacin (Indocin), and piroxicam (Feldene). These common pain relievers do more harm than good. They can bother the GI tract in a number of different ways, says Robert Hoffman, MD, chief of rheumatology at the University Of Miami Miller School Of Medicine. "Gastritis, esophageal reflux disease [heartburn or GERD], and bleeding ulcers are all problems that can develop from NSAIDs." They also destroy the lining of your stomach. According to the National

Digestive Diseases Information Clearinghouse. "Normally the stomach has three defenses against digestive juices: mucus that coats the stomach lining and shields it from stomach acid, the chemical bicarbonate that neutralizes stomach acid, and blood circulation to the stomach lining that aids in cell renewal and repair," the clearinghouse explains. "NSAIDs hinder all of these protective mechanisms, and with the stomach's defenses down, digestive juices can damage the sensitive stomach lining and cause ulcers." Stomach Acid Blockers slow down the production of stomach acid. We need our stomach acid. if your stomach acid is low then food doesn't digest well. This is when you start to experience symptoms such as bloating, belching, bad breath, feeling like skipping meals and yes, heartburn. So guess what? Heartburn is often the under production of stomach acid. Therefore Dietary changes are a MUST. Why keep eating things that upset your stomach anyways? If it's not agreeing with you. This like a kid who has gotten burned by a hot eye on a stove but yet keeps putting their hand on it again and again yet to be burned over and over.  Once you begin this new KETO AIP protocol you will see that when you have eliminated processed foods, refined carbohydrates, sugar and grains just to name a few no more medication will be needed.

## Our digestive system doesn't absorb food, it absorbs nutrients.

For most people, taking a quality probiotic supplement doesn't have any side effects other than higher energy and better digestive health. As a society we have drastically cut back on our consumption of vegetables and of beneficial essential fatty acids ( flax, pumpkin, black current seed oil, dark green leafy vegetables, hemp, chia seeds, fish) such as those found in certain fish (including salmon, mackerel, and herring) and flaxseed. We are consumed with little fiber and an excess of sugar, salt, and processed foods. Stress, changes in the diet, contaminated food, chlorinated water, and numerous other factors can also alter the bacterial flora in the intestinal tract. When you treat the whole person instead of just treating a disease or symptom, an imbalance in the intestinal tract stands out like an elephant in the room. To play it safe, I take a quality probiotic supplement every day.

Probiotics are live bacteria and yeasts that are good for your health, especially your digestive system. Probiotics are often called "good" or "helpful" bacteria because they help keep your gut healthy. Probiotics foods include yogurt, kefir, Kimchi, Sour Pickles ( brined in water and sea salt instead of vinegar) Pickle juice is rich in electrolytes, and has been shown to help relieve exercise-induced muscle cramps., Kombucha, kombucha tea ,Fermented meat, fish, and eggs.

Fixing that unhappy belly by providing the nutrients and amino acids needed to start building a healthy gut lining. Most people simply do not understand how complex the human gastrointestinal system is, and contrary to popular belief, your gut isn't just a food processing and storage depot. Did you know that your gut has so much influence on your health is because it is home to roughly 100,000,000,000,000 (100 trillion) bacteria (approximately 3 pounds worth) that line your intestinal tract. Your gut is the home control center to your digestive system, your nervous system, as well as your immune system.

## 13. Avoid SOY!

Soy not only disrupts hormones by mimicking estrogen in your body but it also causes inflammation,  contributes to leaky gut syndrome and most likely has been genetically modified (GMO). Start reading your labels. You will be surprised how companies will sneak in soy.

Brilliant marketing campaigns have lead you to believe that soy products are healthy but in fact it's completely the opposite. Soy products are not healthy foods. Eating soy frequently can potentially lead to numerous other health issues.

For centuries, Asian people have been consuming fermented soy products such as natto, tempeh, and soy sauce, and enjoying the health benefits. Fermented soy does not wreak havoc on your body like unfermented soy products do.

The issue with soy is most soy today contains something called phytoestrogens, and these phytoestrogens are estrogen mimickers in the body. And so, if you're a male consuming extra estrogen, it's going to give you more feminine characteristics.

If you're a woman consuming foods that increase estrogen levels, it's going to increase your risk of breast cancer, cervical cancer, PCOS (polycystic ovary syndrome) and other hormone imbalance-related disorders.

Many have felt as if they needed a diary substitute since they couldn't tolerate dairy. Actually your body was doing you an even bigger favor.

For starters, some chemicals such as isoflavones, found in soy products like soy milk or edamame, can intercept your thyroid's ability to make hormones if you're not getting enough iodine.

Soybeans are one of the crops that are being genetically modified. Since 1997 GMO soybeans are being used in an increasing number of products.

Dr. Kaayla Daniel, author of The Whole Soy Story, points out thousands of studies linking soy to malnutrition, digestive distress, immune-system breakdown, thyroid dysfunction, cognitive decline, reproductive disorders and infertility—even cancer and heart disease. Here is just a sampling of the health effects that have been linked to soy consumption:

   Breast cancer

   Brain damage

   Infant abnormalities

   Thyroid disorders

Kidney stones

Immune system impairment

Severe, potentially fatal food allergies

Impaired fertility

Danger during pregnancy and nursing

Final thoughts on Soy: Soy is terrible – contains trypsin inhibitors, is a source of xenoestrogens, even if it's organic, and if it's GMO, it also comes with a lot of glyphosate and other pesticide residues. Avoid it like the black plague.

## 14. Invest in a water filter

The water that comes from your sink probably contains chlorine or fluoride (or both)—which can also disrupt the thyroid by interfering with its ability to absorb iodine properly that it needs to produce hormones. I use a Berkey Water Tank.

## 15. Drink plenty of water!

Drinking Water will help your body maintain the Balance of Bodily Fluids. Your body is made up of 60% water. The liquid helps your bodily fluids include digestion, absorption, circulation, creation of saliva, transportation of nutrients, and control of body's temperature. Try to think of water as a necessary nutrient to keep your body working. If your Cells don't maintain enough fluids and electrolytes it can result in muscle fatigue.

## 16. Start eating Fermented Foods

There are incredible health benefits when you start incorporating fermented foods to your diet. Did you know that your gut is the largest component of your immune system? It introduces friendly bacteria into your digestive system that helps to keep illness's at bay and they are rich in live bacteria that help us absorb nutrients along with maintain proper microbiome gut balance. Research has proven that gut health could affect inflammation, allergies and autoimmune disorders in the body as a whole. Around 1,000 different species of bugs live in your gut. We acquire them at birth (initially in the birth canal) and during the early years of childhood.

Your gut has been linked to contributing to weight loss and for overall improvement of numerous symptoms, including depression, anxiety, brain fog, skin problems, hormonal issues, immune weaknesses, digestive problems, and fatigue.

## 17. Avoid Hormones and Antibiotics-

Most Livestock animals that provide meat and dairy products unless they are from an all organic farm are tainted with growth hormones, antibiotics and GMO feed. These chemicals pass through the food chain to us the consumers. Growth hormones can cause opposite sex characteristics in developing children, early puberty, the development of cancer, and infertility. Even scarier is the world is becoming immune to antibiotics and these superbugs. Due from all the constant exposure from our food supply. Our bodies are becoming more resistant to the antibiotics that use to be able to easily treat an infection or a foreign body invader.

## 18. Change your cookware

Reduce Exposure to the Chemical PFOA (Found in Non-Stick Cookware)

Finally, reduce your exposure to PFOA, found in common household products including nonstick cookware and waterproof fabrics. Researchers have found that people with higher levels of PFOA (perfluorooctanoic acid) have a higher incidence of thyroid disease.

Start cooking with cast iron skillets or stainless steel cookware.


## 19. Make your own toothpaste

Fluoride blocks iodine receptors

Did you know that fluoride was Once Prescribed as an Anti-Thyroid Drug?   Up through the 1950s, doctors in Europe and South America prescribed fluoride to reduce thyroid function in patients with over-active thyroids (hyperthyroidism). (Merck Index 1968).   Although fluoride concentrations in tap water are relatively low and are considered "safe" for human consumption, it is not. Fluoride has long-term neurological and hormonal affects.  Fluoride is not an essential nutrient.  It is also that chemical that is commonly found in most toothpaste brands.  There is clear evidence that, when ingested at high doses, fluoride causes neurotoxicity. Fluoride also is understood to interfere with the absorption of iodine, possibly leading to an iodine deficiency and ultimately hypothyroidism.  To benefit your health, use fluoride free tooth or make your own tooth paste.

Oral health is connected with the rest of the body and it's easy to forget where the first step of digestion occurs: Yes, in the mouth!

Why would you continue to use toothpastes that include sodium lauryl phosphate, triclosan, glycerin, fluoride, and other potentially harmful chemicals? Just look at the warning labels on a standard tube of toothpaste!

Did you know that your teeth are living and spongy. The foods we eat, the commercial toothpastes, medications and chemicals from drinks all can suck out the minerals from the teeth causing weakened enamel and leaving us more susceptible to decay and breakdown. I was on a new mission to keep my teeth healthy by using the absolute necessary and needed trace minerals to maintain the upmost dental health plus find a solution that wasn't abrasive, while gently polishing them, and detoxifies while it refreshes. Is there such a thing? I did know that my long history with Mr. Store bought toothpaste was over. Did you know that a tooth powder could whiten your teeth, remove plaque, and not contain any harmful chemicals or questionable additives?

If you haven't already, you should invest in a water filtration system to rid your tap water of fluoride. Do we really know how safe tap water is? Look at the recent events in Flint Michigan! Can you really trust the water companies? Although fluoride concentrations in tap water are relatively low and are considered "safe" for human consumption, it is not. Fluoride has long-term neurological and hormonal affects. Fluoride is not an essential nutrient. It is also that chemical that is commonly found in most toothpaste brands. There is clear evidence that, when ingested at high doses, fluoride causes neurotoxicity. Fluoride also is understood to interfere with the absorption of iodine, possibly leading to an iodine deficiency and ultimately hypothyroidism. To benefit your health, use fluoride free tooth or make your own tooth paste. Get a good water filtration system and purchase a filter for your shower head. We use a Berkefeld brand.

Store bought toothpaste also have other ingredients in it like:

Glycerin is used in almost all toothpastes because it helps create a pasty texture and prevents it from drying out. Although it's non-toxic it coats the teeth just enough to that prevents normal tooth remineralization. Remineralization is a whole-body process and in order for it to happen, the body must have adequate levels of certain nutrients, especially fat soluble vitamins and certain minerals. If you want to stop and reverse Tooth Decay you must add minerals in your diet, add plenty of fat soluble vitamins (A, D, E and K), and your body must be able to absorb vital nutrients. You certainly can't do this by having a coat on your teeth that will prevent absorption.

Sodium Lauryl Sulfate (SLS) is a foaming agent and detergent that is commonly used in toothpaste, shampoo, and other products such as degreaser for car engines. SLS is an estrogen mimicker. It also increases gum inflammation and mouth ulcers. According to a study conducted the Department of Oral Surgery & Oral Medicine in Oslo, Norway, individuals who used a toothpaste containing SLS suffered from more ulcers (canker sores) than those who used an SLS-free toothpaste.

Sweeteners: Sorbitol, sodium saccharin and other artificial sweeteners are often used in toothpaste to improve taste, even though there is no evidence that these sweeteners are beneficial (or even safe) for use in the mouth. Xylitol has shown some positive benefits for oral health in some studies, but it remains a controversial ingredient in toothpaste.

Triclosan: A chemical used in antibacterial soaps and products. Triclosan was recently found to affect proper heart function in a study at University of California Davis and the FDA is currently re-evaluating it for safety in human use.

Let's not forget to mention that many toothpastes also contain artificial colors/dyes or synthetic flavors. I must admit there are several good natural toothpastes out there and I have tried some of them not all but with my tight budget I will make them for pennies on the dollar. My favorite way to brush my teeth is by using tooth powder. Yes, you read this right. Tooth Powder. Here is my recipe that I use. Feel free to adjust the ingredient's based on your own needs. If you have sensitive teeth you might want to skip the baking soda and salt until you can get used to it.

# Homemade Tooth Powder Recipe

(Who would have thought that a toothpaste could be Keto AIP friendly?)

## Ingredients

4 tablespoons Bentonite Clay (make sure it is calcium not Sodium Bentonite Clay)

2 teaspoons baking soda

1 ½ teaspoons finely ground Himalayan sea salt

½ teaspoons clove powder

1 teaspoon ground Ceylon cinnamon

5-10 drops of food grade peppermint essential oil

¾ teaspoons activated charcoal – optional

## Directions

Using a stainless steel or plastic spoon, mix all ingredients in a clean glass jar. To use, add a little to a wet toothbrush and brush as normal.

## Bentonite Clay

Bentonite clay is a gentle cleanser that is rich in minerals which support tooth remineralization. Its detoxifying properties help freshen breath and fight gum disease, while it's adsorptive properties help remove stains from teeth. Make sure to get the food grade natural calcium brand like this one below. This is the brand that I use.

## Baking Soda

Baking soda is a mild abrasive tooth polish that helps mechanically remove stains while other ingredients such as clay and activated charcoal draw them out. It also helps freshen breath.

## Himalayan Sea Salt

Himalayan sea salts such as this one contain 60+ trace minerals that aid in tooth remineralization. Salt is also highly antiseptic, which helps keep bacteria in check.

## Herb & Spices

Spices and herbs such as clove powder, ground cinnamon, and ground mint add flavoring, but they also have astringent properties that support gum health.

## Activated Charcoal

Activated carbon – is made by processing charcoal with oxygen and either calcium chloride or zinc chloride. It was used medicinally by both Hippocrates and the ancient Egyptians, and it is still the poison remedy of choice in modern day emergency rooms. Why? Because it's highly adsorptive, which in plain English means it attracts substances to its surface like a magnet. Like absorptive substances which work like a sponge, adsorptive materials bind with certain compounds and prevent our bodies from using them.

If you're not so hip on using powdered tooth, then here are some more all natural recipes.

## Natural Peppermint Toothpaste

1/2 cup coconut oil

3 Tablespoons of baking soda

15 drops of peppermint food grade essential oil

Melt to soften the coconut oil. Mix in other ingredients and stir well. Place your mixture into small glass jar. Allow it to cool completely. When ready to use just dip toothbrush in and scrape small amount onto bristles.

## Homemade Coconut Oil Toothpaste Recipe

6 tbsp. coconut oil

6 tbsp. baking soda

15-20 drops of a food grade essential oil (peppermint, cinnamon, grapefruit or lemon taste great)

Melt to soften the coconut oil. Mix in other ingredients and stir well. Place your mixture into small glass jar. Allow it to cool completely. When ready to use just dip toothbrush in and scrape small amount onto bristles.

## Homemade Tooth Powder Recipe

**Ingredients**

4 tablespoons calcium Bentonite clay

2 teaspoons baking soda

1 ½ teaspoons finely ground unrefined sea salt

½ teaspoons clove powder

1 teaspoon ground Ceylon cinnamon

5-10 drops of peppermint essential oil

¾ teaspoons activated charcoal –

Directions

Using a stainless steel or plastic spoon, mix all ingredients in a clean glass jar. To use, add a little to a wet toothbrush and brush as normal.

Curious about the dangers of fluoride?

<u>The Fluoride Deception</u>

This is a powerful read and you can purchase pretty much anywhere. The Fluoride Deception documents a powerful connection between big corporations, the U.S. military, and the historic reassurances of fluoride safety provided by the nation's public health establishment. The Fluoride Deception reads like a thriller, but one supported by two hundred pages of source notes, years of investigative reporting, scores of scientist interviews, and archival research in places such as the newly opened files of the Manhattan Project and the Atomic Energy Commission. The book is nothing less than an exhumation of one of the great secret narratives of the industrial era: how a grim workplace poison and the most damaging environmental pollutant of the cold war was added to our drinking water and toothpaste.

## 20. Get some Sleep

If you're not getting enough rest it will cause your body to become suppressed, which will slow your body from healing itself. You need to have a healthy sleep cycle. Many reasons why you may suffer from insomnia, difficulty falling asleep or even staying asleep but nutritional imbalances, environmental toxins, stress, hormonal imbalances and thyroid issues all can play a role in your sleep cycle.

You need to look at your life. Environmental factors, dietary habits, and medical history all play a role in this. There are 5 proven foods that exacerbate insomnia which are caffeine, Nightshades, Alcohol, and Aged, fermented, cured, smoked, and cultured foods, Sugar, Flour, and other Refined Carbohydrates. These foods listed are foods that we discuss in my book. Changing how you eat is one of the most powerful and important ways to change your brain chemistry. Always keep a food journal and write down any symptoms. Sometimes you might feel the effects of what you've eaten until hours later. Discovering what triggers your insomnia will give you that peace of mind and a sound, restful good night's sleep that you've been longing for.

## 21. Avoid caffeine

Caffeine adds stress to your adrenal glands and the endocrine system. Caffeine will stimulate you adrenals causing them to adrenaline and cortisol in the exact same way as they do during a 'fight or flight' reaction. Caffeine gives you a false boost in energy before the fall to fatigue.

Your thyroid is very sensitive to stimulants. It only confuses your already overworked system.

If you must have coffee, try to limit it to one cup of coffee a day.

As for caffeinated soda, this beverage is a loaded with empty calories, a crazy amount of sugar and then top if off with the caffeine. You can purchase soda water without sodium and squeeze a lemon or lime into it.

## 22. Avoid Sugary Foods

Eating sugar is making your adrenal glands work harder. Stop indirectly making your adrenal gland producing extra cortisol to fight the excess sugar.

There's no way to sugarcoat the truth — Americans are eating more sugar than ever before. Researchers from the University of North Carolina at Chapel Hill determined that, on average, Americans are consuming 83 more calories per day from caloric sweeteners than they did in 1977. And those extra 83 calories a day turn into a whopping 2,490 calories per month.

Sugar addiction is nothing to joke about. Once you're hooked, cravings can be very hard to fight against, leading you down a never ending movement towards obesity and other health problems. Studies are showing that in some people and animals, the brain can react to sugar very much like it can to drugs and alcohol. That's why when you initially cut added sugars from your diet, you might feel deprived for a few days. "When your body is overloaded with waste, you feel more uncomfortable when not eating that food," Fuhrman says. "It's like stopping coffee."

Besides research showing that amazing not-so-innocent sweet tooth could be doing serious damage to your health, leading to weight gain, high blood pressure and cholesterol levels and an increased risk for diabetes. Matter of a fact, Dr. Joel Fuhrman, author of The End of Dieting, says eating too much sugar should be considered just as dangerous as smoking cigarettes. "A diet with sugar and high glycemic index foods promotes all the leading causes of death in America," he says. "I don't see value in cutting out sugar for a few days and then going back to eating it, but I do see value in cutting it out permanently." Don't think for one moment that artificial sweeteners are better. Artificial sweeteners are synthetic sugar substitutes. "Artificial sweeteners are not risk-free," said Brian Hoffmann, assistant professor in the Department of Biomedical Engineering at the Medical College of Wisconsin. Artificial sweeteners appear to contribute to metabolic disorders by altering the activity of certain genes responsible for the breakdown of macromolecules such as fats and proteins, Hoffmann said. This is different from normal sugars, which contribute to cardiovascular disease through insulin resistance and by damaging the cells lining the body's blood vessels.


## 23. READ food labels

Stay away from fake, made in a lab, made by man, processed or artificial foods aka Frankenstein foods meaning they are not real. Remember if it can sit on the shelf for a long time, it certainly can sit in your body the same way.

## 24. Are you on a medication that makes you gain weight?

Certain medications, notably steroids, and also some antidepressants, antipsychotics, high blood pressure drugs, allergy medication, birth control, and seizure medications has been linked to adding the extra lbs. to your waistline. Keep in mind we are all different not everybody will experience the same side effects if any with medications.

Don't ever stop taking any medications without first consulting your doctor. You're on that medication for a reason and it just may be critical to your health. Please always consult with your doctor so they can try to help you figure out what's going on but be honest. Don't go into the doctor's office saying your gaining weight and you can't figure it out knowing you had that diet coke & Twinkie for breakfast!

## 25. *Water Boosts Metabolism*

I've already covered this but let me go over it again. Lots of people don't realize the true importance of drinking enough water every day and how it can impact both your health and your weight loss efforts. "Water's involved in every type of cellular process in your body, and when you're dehydrated, everything runs less efficiently.  It slows down your metabolism.

Your metabolism is basically a series of chemical reactions that take place in your body. Staying hydrated keeps those chemical reactions moving smoothly. If you are even slightly dehydrated that will affect your metabolism.

Aim for at least 100 ounces a day –
especially in the first couple of weeks until
your body adjusts or half your body weight in
ounces.

## 26. Keeping your Blood Sugar in Check

Low GI (glycemic index)/ Low Carb diets are
based on the principles of balancing your
blood sugar. The reason for keeping your
blood sugar in check is to not have your
blood sugar and insulin levels to rise to fast
and high. This roller coaster of blood sugar
highs and lows will activate your stress
hormones and are catabolic to our tissues
including the gut lining, lungs and brain. Your
body is in one of two states throughout the
day. You're either in an anabolic state or a
catabolic state. If your body is in a constant
catabolic state the protective barriers will
become worn down over time and it over
activates the immune system creating chaos

where the body gets confused and attacks itself and wasting away as is the case with Hashimoto's or basically any autoimmune condition. Three things also can contribute to a catabolic state. Not working out smart. Not eating the right food. Not getting enough rest. If you are in a catabolic state you take the change of your body cannibalizing muscle. If you're in an anabolic state is it means that you're exercising correctly, you're eating the right foods and you are getting plenty of rest.  Remember you can be creating more cortisol to store in your mid-section by over exercising. You want to stimulate the metabolism, not annihilate it.  The easiest way to balance blood sugar and remain in an anabolic state is to eliminate processed carbohydrates and sugar, plan meals around protein and healthy fats then load up your plate with low carb/low GI.


## 27. Eat more Nutrient Dense Foods

Think about what you're putting in your body. Either you're fighting disease or feeding disease. You must get a concept of nutrient density. Many of the foods we tend to eat, block nutrients from being absorbed. Gluten, dairy and soy products create inflammation in the digestive tract. In ancient times grains were prepared by soaking, sprouting and fermenting but that tradition in making them been long forgotten with our fast-paced culture. If you have inflammation in the digestive system undigested proteins leak into the blood stream creating a heightened immune reaction that often makes your thyroid issues worse and can lead to a leaky gut which causes other problems.

## 28. Reduce your inflammation

Chronic inflammation can spread and have more harmful effects than just one area in your body. Your body can experience things like higher blood pressure , allergies, create autoimmune issues, experience joint pain, cause heart problems, harmful swelling, bone loss, it can lower your iron levels and it just have a negative impact on your entire well-being. Did you know that chronic inflammation can also raise your reverse T3, which means this might be the reason why your hypothyroidism was created in the 1st place. We must get the inflammation under control. Cut out foods like gluten, sugar, refined carbs, fake foods, soy, and vegetable oils and add in fresh whole fruits, healthy fats and fiber. Start creating your own body lotions and cleaning supplies.

## 29. Relieve Your Stress

Many of us find ourselves in this cycle of so much responsibility that at times it seems impossible to manage. We are over worked and the chronic stress is breaking us down. Chronis stress keeps our cortisol levels elevated. If our cortisol levels are staying elevated, it begins to interfere with many other areas of our body which are the immune system, digestion, sleep, and even the ability to produce other essential hormones such as estrogen, progesterone, testosterone, and YES you named it last but not least our THYROID which can cause an autoimmune reaction. Do you see the cycle?

We must try to begin to tackle our stress and start to manage it.

Stress not only effects your immune system but by revving up your immune system, it begins to produces a wave of inflammation.

Let's face it your immune system needs a long vacation from all the stress you've put it through. Just enough for a fighting chance to get back on track.....

Take a walk, read a book, take a relaxing Epsom salt bath, start a yoga class, meditate, walk your dog. The key is to figure out what works for you and relaxes you.

I want to arm you with tools that you need to help you start managing your condition.

You have the power to make a difference in your life. You've always had the power. No one can force you to become more aware of what you put on your body and what you put in your body. What you eat is just as important as what you put on your body. Adjusting your life, reading labels and catering to your specific health needs isn't easy but it will benefit you in the long run. This is one of the smartest decisions that you can make. Not only will you start to look and feel better but think of the medical cost that you could be saving your future self.

We need to be kind to ourselves. Give our bodies a fighting chance. If you constantly feed your body crap then you are making it susceptible to inflammation, viruses and disease. I want to help you become successful in your healthy journey by applying the empowering techniques many of my blogs have to offer.

## 30. Always Choose Organic*

Foods that are not organic grown have been sprayed with pesticides, herbicides, insecticides and fungicides and could possibly be genetically modified. This can add to the toxic build up on your lymph nodes.

### PESTICIDE WASH AND VEGETABLE CLEANER

When you are trying to have an AIP Keto friendly kitchen you want to try to remove all pesticides, Genetically Modified Organisms (GMO's), and other unwanted chemicals from your diets. Whenever it's possible try to opt for organic and non GMO fruit/vegetables. Sometimes it's just not possible to purchase organic produce so here is a recipe that can help you minimize the consumption of unwanted chemicals. Keep in mind that you should always try to purchase organic fruits/vegetable is you because not all I pesticides can be removed from washing.

In a your sink, a washing basin or large bowl, make a solution of 1 part white vinegar & 3 parts room temperature filtered water. Research has shown that a 3 part water to 1 part vinegar solution is most effective, removing 98% of contaminants.

The EPA's Safe Drinking Water Act (1974) only regulates 91 of the over 60,000 chemicals used in the United States. The tap water of at least 41 million Americans has been found to contain a wide range of pharmaceuticals and over the counter medications, caused by the combination of every medication user's excretory system and a flush of the toilet.

Next place your room temperature fruits and vegetables into the wash mixture. Try to keep the solution and your fruit/vegetables near the same temperature, where you can reduce the risk of shock to certain soft-skinned fruits and vegetables. Temperature shock can cause pores in the skins to intake more of the dirty water, and thus more of the chemicals you are trying to remove.

Allow the fruits and vegetables to soak for ten minutes.

Air dry on a towel or washed counter space. I always like to give mine an extra rinse before eating. Don't forget to label with a black permanent marker.

# HOMEMADE SPRAY PESTICIDE WASH

Add 1 Tbsp. of fresh Lemon Juice, 2 Tbsp. of distilled White Vinegar and 1 Cup of Filtered Water to a BPA free spray bottle.

Tighten the lid and give it a good shake.

Don't be shy about spraying this wash on your produce and rub the mixture for 20-30 seconds by hand or use a good vegetable brush (on hard produce such as tomatoes, potatoes or apples). Afterwards rinse well with again clean filtered water.

| DIRTY DOZEN™ Buy These Organic | | CLEAN 15™ Lowest in Pesticides | |
|---|---|---|---|
| WORST | 1 Celery | BEST | 1 Onions |
| | 2 Peaches | | 2 Avocado |
| | 3 Strawberries | | 3 Sweet Corn |
| | 4 Apples | | 4 Pineapple |
| | 5 Blueberries | | 5 Mangos |
| | 6 Nectarines | | 6 Sweet Peas |
| | 7 Bell Peppers | | 7 Asparagus |
| | 8 Spinach | | 8 Kiwi |
| | 9 Cherries | | 9 Cabbage |
| | 10 Kale/Collard Greens | | 10 Eggplant |
| | 11 Potatoes | | 11 Cantaloupe |
| | 12 Grapes (Imported) | | 12 Watermelon |
| | | | 13 Grapefruit |
| | | | 14 Sweet Potato |
| | | | 15 Honeydew Melon |

## 32. Address Hormonal imbalances

Why it is that one person can eat all they want and never gain an inch, while someone else gains weight just looking at food? The fact is some people are wired to simply burn fat better than others. There are sneaky little things in your body that can halt your weight loss success.

Where you store your body fat isn't a topic most of us women like to discuss but I feel it is one that will enlighten you and help you more on your journey to a better healthier you.

After researching many days on this topic, I've found that where your body stores fat is hint to what is going on with you internally with your hormones. As our hormone levels change with age, pregnancy, exercise, eating habits, or other life events, fat adjusts itself to our every changing hormonal events and places itself in different area's in our body. Our hormones have a direct impact on how much body fat we store and where it is stored on our bodies. Wouldn't it be wonderful to know what approach to take to fix those thunder thighs or that muffin top? Now even with this information it's just a stepping stone of knowledge to better equip you a healthier you. This completely changes how you and what you should be eating.

So what exactly does it mean to have fat stored in certain areas of your body and not others?

Every cell in our body responds to the foods we eat, the products we put on our bodies and the household chemicals that we come in contact with every day. Although some of us were born with the predisposition genetics as our parents that gives us our hair color, eye color, height and if we are pear shaped, apple shaped, straight or hourglass this doesn't mean we can't win the battle when it comes to our hormones. Our hormones have a direct impact on every major system in our body. Remember our bodies love balance. Everything has a domino effect so we have to try to figure-out that balance in what our individual body needs are. Whether it be the more fiber, fixing our gut, helping our skin get more moisture, speeding up our metabolism so we can get out of that fat storage mode and into the fat burning mode.

Love handles/belly: Love handles often means that you are way too stressed out and when you're stressed out it raises your cortisol levels. It could also be an indicator that you might have adrenal fatigue. Cortisol adds fat around my mid-section. You are eating too much sugar where you become insulin resistant. If your body is in constant elevated levels of insulin (a hormone that regulates the metabolism of carbohydrates in the bloodstream) it will accumulate around your mid-section. A lack of sleep also may lead to metabolic issues and help encourage those love handles. It also could mean you have elevated estrogen levels and more insulin production. So what do you need to do? Stop eating crap, those processed carbs and avoid sugar, even the fake sugars which are even more horrible for you. You should also go easy on the exercise, sometimes if you exercise more it adds more cortisol to your body so you are fighting a losing battle, try yoga, more sleep, meditation, Pilates, planks, lifting weights and walking are good ways to start. Don't forget fat gained around the waist is dangerous in terms of it increases the risk of heart disease, diabetes and other chronic diseases.

Thighs: Sometimes it's our genetic bone structure that was passed down from our parents that gives us more hips or fatter thighs than the next person and other times it can mean that we have elevated estrogen levels. This is the female sex hormone. Thigh fat is a little harder to burn off than belly fat. You can also have fluid retention in your thighs. So many think that fluid retention only takes place only in the abdomen but that isn't true It actually occurs all over your body. So what do you need to do? Start drinking your daily needed allowance of water. Your body weight and divide it by two. That's the least amount of water to drink per day and please don't drink it all in one sitting. There is a think called water toxicity and it will kill you. Space out your water consumption. Choose better skin care products in my blog 21 Successful Tips on Clean Beauty Swaps. I share with your skin care products are healthier. You want to avoid chemicals such as BPA (that can be found in plastic containers, water bottles and pretty much anything plastic unless it states BPA FREE), parabens or phthalates. Your food should be 100% organic and you most defiantly should be avoiding all soy products like the black plague. Let's not forget that getting in a good night's sleep will also help to improve your estrogen levels.

Back of Arms: This could mean that you have lower testosterone levels as well as an excess insulin. Women do have a small amount of testosterone in our adrenal glands and ovaries although this is thought as a male hormone. Start eating more avocados, as in healthy fats and fatty fish such as salmon can help improve this area. Try to avoid all red meat and all dairy products. Start trying to lift some weights. Building muscle through weight lifting can and may also increase testosterone levels.

Upper Back: This could mean you have lower levels of Thyroxine and higher levels of insulin. Thyroxine is a thyroid hormone that plays a role with your metabolism and calorie burning rate and this hormone is secreted into our bloodstream. You can help boost your thyroxine naturally by eating foods such as shellfish, seafood and cruciferous vegetables, avoiding gluten and soy, and increasing healthy fat intake.

Our metabolism does not decide to burn or store body fat based on calories. It makes these decisions based on the hormones those calories trigger. That is why the quality of calories matters so much…. higher-quality calories trigger body-fat-burning hormones while low-quality calories trigger body-fat-storing hormones.

Body fat is important necessity for life. It is our source of energy and it stores some much needed nutrients, a major ingredient in brain tissue. Moreover, it provides a padding to protect internal organs and insulates the body against the cold. But yet, getting too fat (more than 30 percent body fat in females and 25 percent in males) can be dangerous and is associated with increased risk of disease and premature death, regardless of where the fat is stored in the body. As an American society, we are tipping the scales to the point that obesity is now a national health epidemic.

Think about this each time you eat, hormones are released into your body and the type of calories consumed (i.e. fat, carbohydrates or protein) determines which hormones are released and where it is placed throughout your body. The only way to achieve your goal is to start eating to cater to your body's specific needs. Along with proper exercise. I know for a fact that if you put forth the effort this can be attainable. There are no shortcuts.

## 33. Help out your digestion process

Digestion is the chemical and mechanical breakdown of food. The goal of your digestion process is to reduce the food to molecules so tiny that the nutrients can be absorbed and used by your cells and turned into fuel for your body, otherwise known as, Adenosine Triphosphate (ATP).

Every single cell that makes up every single tissue that makes up every single organ depends on the body's digestive system to provide the necessary nutrients it needs to keep on functioning.

A few ways you can help your digestion process is to reduce your stress, chew your food where the enzymes can be properly activated, stay hydrated so that your body can properly transport nutrients through your digestive tract and also limit the liquids at mealtime to avoid diluting your gastric juices. Try consuming fermented foods and last but not least try walking after a meal. This helps to reduce stress but also it stimulates the muscle contractions necessary for digestion.

# Keto AIP Foods to Eat and What to Avoid

This will be a big adjustment to your life and I 'm not going to sugar coat it. The 1st few days or even the 1st few weeks might be hard because you won't be consuming any sugar, bad carbs, processed foods, caffeine, Nightshades, Eggs, Grains (gluten), Dairy, Legumes, Corn, Soy and lectins.  This book is also unlike any other traditional keto guides. In this book, you're not going to focus on macros, calories, or follow strict rules.

Instead, I want you to use the resources that is given and learn how to use the proper portion sizes. Feeling the freedom of focusing on what you can eat and learn what feels right for your body and your health.

We are all individuals and each one of us are unique with our own metabolic and nutrition efficiency needs. We must begin to listen, become accountable and understand where our bodies are struggling to begin weight-loss and becoming healthier. There is no secret magical pill. It does take discipline, commitment and action. I cannot, no matter how hard I try do growth work for YOU. This is your choice to decide to better your life and become healthy. Eating well isn't boring nor bland. Once you learn how to eat to nourish your body you are going to feel so much better.

How do you know if you eating the proper portion sizes? Keto AIP is 10 % low GI carbs, 20% protein and 70% fats but you see we aren't following any "rules". We are learning proper portion sizes which are different with Keto AIP.

When you go to eat imagine a line the divides the plate in half which will make the plate

into two parts Then imagine half of one side
another line dividing that in to two sections.
The large section is where you are going to
fill up with low GI vegetables.


You can purchase food portion control plates
off of amazon. That are 3 tiered.  For
instance, here is a sample plate. Please
ignore the grain image. I wanted to simply
share what a 3 tier plate looks like.

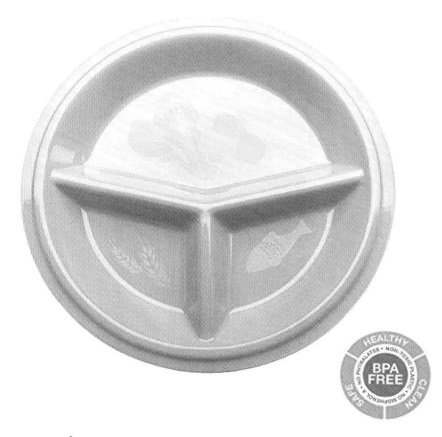

# *BEING PREPARED IS KEY TO SUCCESS*

If you've been told that Keto AIP is just like the Atkins plan, then you've been misguided. This plan is low amounts of good quality protein, high amounts of good fats and plenty of low GI organic vegetables.

You must meal prep, pack snacks and have things readily available at your fingertips. Planning ahead and being prepared will be the key to your success. This is your journey and I know you can do this.

I love using these containers to help me meal prep and I also use mason jars.

# What You Can Eat: The YES:

You really have unlimited options of things you can eat and always try to be created with your food. If you find that you don't like any of the recipes given, then create your own. This is your journey. For instance, Salmon, there are hundreds upon hundreds of great recipes for salmon. All you have to do is take what is on the approved list and create from there. I know there are a so many ways you can eat anything that I have listed. This isn't about me, it's about you but I have shared with you so many recipes that I find to be wonderfully delicious and my palate really enjoys. Not only my palate but they tend to help my body thrive and heal.

Grass fed meats, nitrate free and uncured turkey bacon, nitrate free and uncured bacon, bison, pasteurized-organic-grass-fed poultry, duck, lamb, wild caught fatty fish, game meats, ground pork, anchovies, cod, perch, sardines, tuna, shrimp and trout.

***Always buy wild-caught fish never farmed seafood***

***Always buy organic and local produce if possible***

Avocado, Asparagus, artichokes, celery, beets, mustard greens, mushrooms, endive, Brussels sprouts, cabbage, cauliflower, bok choy, broccoli, cucumber (seeds and skin removed), Jamaica, lettuce, spinach, beets, leeks, blueberries, onions, garlic, EVOO, avocado oil, MCT oil, unrefined organic coconut oil, avocado, olives, Coconuts, Chia, flax and hemp seeds. full fat coconut milk, kumbucha, sparkling water, coconut milk kefir, coconut milk yogurt, water kefir, pink Himalayan salt, cinnamon, garlic, lemon balm, basil, chamomile, chives, cloves, coriander, dill weed, ginger, garlic, lavender, horseradish, oregano leaves, parsley, rosemary, saffron, sage, turmeric and thyme. Fermented vegetables, green tea, herbal teas, bone broth, fish broth, and vegetable broths. coconut butter, duck fat, lard, bacon fat, tallow, collagen peptides, gelatin, organic apple cider vinegar, kelp noodles, matcha powder, coconut amino's, red boat fish sauce, coconut flour, lemon, limes, broccoli rabe, collard greens, swiss chard, turnip greens, unsweetened shredded coconut. Romaine, red & green leaf lettuce, kohlrabi, spinach, butter lettuce, parsley, fennel, and seaweed/sea vegetables, parsley, parsnips, mint.

The only exceptions are vinegars with added sugar, or malt vinegar, which generally contains gluten.

You can have squash, pumpkins, and zucchini but you must remove the seeds because they are full of lectins.

Chia, flax and hemp are very low in overall lectins and their nutritional benefits (essential fats, fiber, anti-oxidants and complete protein) outweigh any small amount of lectin that they may have in them.

# The NO's:

No sugar, Artificial sweeteners, coffee, caffeine products, chocolate, peppers, eggplant, green beans, peas or seed based spices like Anise Seed, Annatto Seed, Black Caraway, Celery Seed, Coriander Seed, Cumin, Dill Seed, Fennel Seed, Fenugreek, Mustard Seed, Nutmeg, Poppy Seed, Sesame Seed, no quinoa, no NIGHTSHADES like Ashwagandha, Capsicums, Potatoes, Tomatoes, Tomatillos, Peppers (of any kind), Cocona, Garden Huckleberries, Kutjera, Naranjillas, Pepinos, Pimentos, Tamarillos, Eggplants/aubergines, Goji berries, Cape Gooseberries, Cayenne pepper, Paprika spice, Chili powder, Red Pepper Flakes, Chili Pepper Flakes, Curry spice powder, Garam Masala spice, Most spice blends, Paleo ketchup, Curry Powder, Red Pepper, Chinese Five-Spice Powder, Steak Seasoning, No fruit, no roots or tubers, no Inflammatory oils, okra, mushrooms,

No vinegars with added sugar, or malt vinegar, which generally contains gluten.

No nuts like Almonds, Brazil Nuts, Hazelnuts, Macadamias, Pecans, Pine Nuts, Pistachios, Pumpkin Seeds, Sesame Seeds, Sunflower Seeds, no seeds except for chia, flax or hemp. No dairy, grains, gluten. NO EGGS, no processed foods. No fermented soy, no food additives, no algae, chlorella or spirulina , no butter, no ghee, oats, corn, dairy, soy, eggs, sugar, tomatoes, all peppers- hot peppers, paprika, chili peppers and sweet peppers, No ashwaganda, goji berries, goose berries, ground cherries, any type of fruit other than blueberries, nutmeg, cayenne pepper, guar gum, all beans, peanuts, avoid NSAIDS, no , no Beans & Legumes like Garbanzo Beans, Black Beans, Kidney Beans, Mung Beans, Lima Beans, Black-Eyed Peas, Lentils, Snow Peas, Sugar Snap Peas, Peanuts, Soybeans, Tofu, Soymilk, White Beans, Pinto Beans, Fava

Beans, Red Beans, no corn, no rice, No DAIRY like Milk, cheese, Ice Cream, Frozen Yogurt, Yogurt, Cream, Sour Cream, Dairy Kefir, no wheat or barley, Emulsifiers / Thickeners

## Soups

These soups can be modified to your liking. For example, If you can't tolerate onions and the recipe calls for onions, just omit the onions or replace it with another approved item on the list that you do like. Not all the recipes calls for coconut milk either. If you don't like coconut milk and the recipe does call for coconut milk then simply omit it and replace it with more broth or nothing. Not everyone will like everything that is in some of the recipes. If you find a recipe that has onions or something you don't like, omit it or simply replace it with another approved item on the list.

# Eating has never been simplier.

1st

Just start with a soup base.

Water, chicken stock, fish stock, beef stock or vegetable stock.

2nd

Pick your approved healthy Fat oil's from the list

 EVOO, avocado oil, MCT oil, unrefined organic coconut oil, coconut butter, duck fat, lard, bacon fat, tallow

3rd

Pick your approved vegetables/fruit from the list

***Always buy organic produce if possible and buying local-organic is a major plus but not everyone has time to go to their local farm markets ***

Avocado, Asparagus, artichokes, celery, beets, mustard greens, mushrooms, endive, Brussels sprouts, cabbage, cauliflower, bok choy, broccoli, cucumber ( seeds and skin removed), Jamaica, lettuce, spinach, beets, leeks, onions, garlic, avocado, olives, Coconuts, Romaine, celery, red & green leaf lettuce, kohlrabi, spinach, butter lettuce, fennel, and seaweed/sea vegetables, parsnips, lemon, limes, broccoli rabe, collard greens, swiss chard, turnip greens, kelp noodles, blueberries

You can have squash, pumpkins, and zucchini but you must remove the seeds because the seeds are full of lectins.

**Fermented vegetables you want to purchase fermented foods but try to find ones with organic ingredients, no sugars added, made with salt not vinegar and they are unpasteurized. ***

4ᵗʰ If you want meat pick an approved meat from the list. You don't have to have meat in your dish this is an option. Personally, I can never eat meat again and be happy. I am not a big meat eating fan but I do occasionally eat poultry products and occasional turkey bacon. My family are big meat eaters. These recipes with meat have been tried on my family members and they really have enjoyed them.

Try to always purchase grass-fed, no hormones or antibiotics , wild, nitrate free uncured and pastured when you can. You will also  get more health benefits from organic, free-range, grass-fed, humanely raised poultry and meats.

Grass fed meats, nitrate free and uncured turkey bacon, nitrate free and uncured bacon, bison, grass-fed beef, no hormones or antibiotics added poultry, duck, lamb, wild caught fatty fish like salmon, cod, haddock, game meats, ground pork, anchovies, cod, perch, sardines, tuna, trout, scallops, clams, halibut, perch, shrimp and trout.

***Always buy wild-caught fish never farmed***

5th approved herbs and Spices

Pink Himalayan salt , cinnamon, garlic, lemon balm, basil, chamomile, chives, cloves, coriander, dill weed, ginger, lavender, horseradish,  oregano leaves, parsley, rosemary, saffron, sage, turmeric, mint, cilantro and thyme

**other- full fat coconut milk, sparkling water, green tea, herbal teas, collagen peptides, gelatin, organic apple cider vinegar, matcha tea powder, coconut amino's, red boat fish sauce, coconut flour

Water kefir, Coconut kefir, Coconut yogurt, Kombucha (make sure you buy or make ones with live cultures and without additives or extra sugar**

Vinegars (including apple cider, coconut water vinegar, red wine,

white wine, balsamic)

Chia, flax and hemp are very low in overall lectins and their nutritional benefits (essential fats, fiber, anti-oxidants and complete protein) outweigh any small amount of lectin that they may have in them.

## Fish Broth (Stock)*

Homemade stock sometimes can resemble a jelly like subtance after being refrigerated. This Stock gelatine has numerous health benefits like idodine, gelatine, calcium, healthy fats and electrolytes that include boosting your immunity and improving digestion. Bone broth is such an exceptional superfood. You can store it up to 2 weeks in the  refrigerator or freeze it in ice cube trays where I find it really easy to transfer the frozen cubes of broth to a resealable freezer bag where they will keep for 6 months. If you freeze a it in cubes just add a cube to a cup of warm water and it will dissolve. This will give you a fresh cup of stock to drink!

2 tablespoons coconut oil

2 celery stalks roughly chopped

2 onions roughly chopped (omit the onions if they don't agree with you)

1 carrots roughly, chopped

3 fish carcasses such as Snapper, Barramundi, or Kingfish (whole, non-oily)

4 slices of ginger

3 tablespoons raw apple cider vinegar

5 sprigs thyme

5 sprigs flat-leaf parsley

1 dried bay leaf

12 cups filtered water

Instructions

Place the fish head or carcass into a large pot with 12 cups of cold water.

Bring to a boil and pour out the water.

Refill the pot with fresh water and  add all the ingridents together.

Simmer with the lid on for around 4 hours.

After done allow to cook and strain the ingridents out. Ladel into mason jars with a tightly sealed lid for the refrigerator or in ice cube to freeze for later use.


## Bone Broth (stock) *

Ingredients

2 pounds bones ( chicken or beef)

1 medium carrot, roughly chopped

1 stick celery, roughly chopped

2 bay leaves

Sprigs of fresh herbs: parsley, rosemary, thyme, oregano, chives

1 tablespoon dried porcini mushrooms ( optional )

1 tablespoon Himalyan sea salt

1 teaspoon apple cider vinegar

12 cups filtered water

Instructions

Place everything into a large pot with the 12 cups of cold water.

Bring to a boil and simmer with the lid on for around 4 hours.

After done allow to cook and strain the ingridents out. Ladel into mason jars with a tightly sealed lid for the refrigerator or in ice cube to freeze for later use.

## Gut-Healing Vegetable Broth*

12 cups filtered water

1 tbsp. coconut oil

1 red onion, peeled and cut in half

1 garlic bulb, peeled and chopped

1 thumb-sized piece of ginger roughly chopped

2 cups of watercress

3-4 cup mixed chopped vegetables and peelings I used carrot peelings, red cabbage, fresh mushrooms, leeks and celery

1/2 cup dried shiitake mushrooms

1/4 of a cup dried wakame seaweed

2 tbsp. ground turmeric

1 tbsp. organic apple cider vinegar

A bunch of fresh parsley

Simply add everything to a large pot. Bring to a boil then simmer, with the lid on, for about an hour.

Once everything has been cooked down, strain the liquid into a large bowl.

After done allow to cook and strain the ingridents out. Ladel into mason jars with a tightly sealed lid for the refrigerator or in ice cube to freeze for later use.


## Bacon Soup (with Broccoli and Asparagus)*

1/2 lb of nitrate free, uncured bacon, diced, plus a couple   strips for garnish

1 small organic onion, peeled and diced

4 cloves organic garlic, peeled and minced

1.5 pounds of organic broccoli, cut into florets, stems dicarded

1.5 pounds of asparagus, roughly chopped, woody ends removed and discarded

4 cups chicken broth

Himalayan sea salt to taste

Over medium heat, brown the bacon until crispy in a stock pot. Add the onions and garlic to the bacon fat and saute for about 2 minutes, stirring often. Next put in the vegetables along with the chicken broth to stock pot. Allow the mixture to come to a boil and then reduce over medium low where it can simmer for about 20 minutes, or until vegetables are tender. Once the vegtables are tender. Allow to cool for about 10 minutes off the hot eye. Carefully put the soup in a blender in batches and blend until smooth. Becareful the mixture may still be warm to hot. Season with himalayan sea salt to taste. Or you can use an immersion blender while the soup is still in the stock pot. Ladle into bowl and enjoy!

## Creamless Cream of Asparagus Soup*

2 tablespoons extra-virgin olive oil, coconut oil or avocado oil

1 organic onion, peeled and diced

1 organic stalk of celery, chopped, ends discarded

1 clove of organic garlic, peeled and minced

3 cups asparagus, roughly chopped into 1 inch pieces, woody ends removed and discarded

5 cups of chicken stock or vegetable stock

1 teaspoon freshly squeezed lemon juice

Himalayan sea salt to taste

Over medium-high heat, Saute the onions, garlic and celery until the onions are soft and translucent,stirring often. Next the asparagus and allow to cook an additional 2 minutes. Add the stock and turn the eye down to allow the soup to simmer for 15 minutes or until the vegetables have become soft. Once the vegtables are tender. Allow to cool for about 10 minutes off the hot eye. Carefully put the soup in batches in a blender and blend until smooth. Becareful the mixture may still be warm to hot. After it is pureed place the soup back in the pot and add the lemon juice. Season with himalayan sea salt to taste. Or you can use an immersion blender while the soup is still in the stock pot. Ladle into bowl and enjoy!

## Asparagus Soup with Creamy Coconut Milk*

1 lb. asparagus, roughly chopped into 1 inch pieces, woody ends removed and discarded

2 large onions, organic onion, peeled and diced

1 Tablespoon extra-virgin olive oil, coconut oil or avocado oil

3 cups bone broth, chicken stock or vegetable stock

2 tsp. organic garlic, peeled and minced

1 tsp. ginger, peeled and minced

1/4 tsp. dried rosemary

1 1/2 cups full fat coconut milk

Himalayan sea salt to taste

Over medium-high heat, Sauté the onions, garlic and ginger until the onions are soft and translucent, stirring often. Next the asparagus and rosemary allow to cook an additional 2 minutes. Add the stock and turn the eye down to allow the soup to simmer for 15 minutes or until the vegetables have become soft. Once the vegetables are tender. Allow to cool for about 10 minutes off the hot eye. Carefully put the soup in batches in a blender and blend until smooth. Be careful the mixture may still be warm to hot. After it is pureed add the coconut milk and combine. Season with Himalayan sea salt to taste. Or you can use an immersion blender while the soup is still in the stock pot. Ladle into bowl and enjoy!

## Roasted Butternut Squash Soup*

1 large butternut squash, peeled, seeds discarded and diced into bite size 1 inch squares

3 organic stalks of celery, chopped, ends discarded

1 large organic onion, peeled and diced

5 cloves of organic garlic, peeled and minced

6 sage leaves

6 sprigs of thyme

1 sprig of rosemary

Himalayan sea salt to taste

2 tablespoon extra-virgin olive oil, coconut oil or avocado oil

3.5 cups bone broth, chicken stock or vegetable stock

Himalayan sea salt to taste

Preheat the oven to 350 F. Place everything in a bowl and mix well until combined except the stock. Next lay the mixture on a large roasting pan. Allow to roast for 1 hour and 15 minutes.

After the vegetables and herbs have roasted and are tender. Discard the stems from the herbs. Using my thumb and index finger I will glide my two fingers across the herbs pulling it off the stem. Place the entire mixture along with the broth in a large stock pot. Using an immersion blender blend until smooth. Or you can use a blender and blend in batches and add to the stock pot in batches. Simmer on low for 10 additional minutes. Season with Himalayan sea salt to taste. Ladle into bowl and enjoy!


## Creamy Bacon and Asparagus Soup*

1 lb. asparagus, roughly chopped into 1 inch pieces, woody ends removed and discarded

1 organic onion, peeled and diced

5 slices of nitrate free and uncured bacon or turkey bacon, cut into bite size pieces

3 cups bone broth, chicken stock or vegetable stock

3 tablespoons extra-virgin olive oil, coconut oil or avocado oil

Himalayan sea salt to taste

Over medium heat, brown the bacon until crispy in a stock pot. (If you are using turkey bacon you must add 3 tablespoons of oil.) Remove the bacon to a plate with a paper towel to catch the grease off the bacon. Leave the bacon grease in the pot. Add the onions and asparagus to the bacon fat and sauté until the onions are soft and translucent, stirring often. Add the broth and using an immersion blender, blend until smooth or you can use a blender and blend in batches and add to the stock pot in batches. Simmer on low for 10 additional minutes. Season with Himalayan sea salt to taste. Ladle into bowl and enjoy!

## Mint Avocado Chilled Soup*

1 medium ripe avocado, cut in half, seed discarded and flesh scooped out

2 organic romaine lettuce leaves

1 cup full fat coconut milk, chilled

1 Tablespoon fresh lime juice

20 fresh mint leaves

Himalayan sea Salt to taste

Place all the ingredients into a blender and combine well. The soup should be thick but not too thick to blend.

Chill in fridge for 5-10 minutes and serve.


## Chilled Blueberry-Rosemary Soup*

3 Cups fresh organic blueberries

1 can full-fat coconut milk, chilled

1/8 tsp fresh rosemary, minced

1/4 tsp Ceylon cinnamon

1 Tablespoon organic apple cider vinegar

1 Tablespoon fresh lemon juice

Himalayan sea salt to taste

In a stock pot place the coconut milk with rosemary, salt, cinnamon, apple cider vinegar, lemon juice, and blueberries. Allow them to simmer for 8-10 minutes.

Remove from the eye and allow the mixture to cool to room temperature. You can either use an immersion blend or add the mixture in batches to your regular blender until its smooth. Ladle into bowls and enjoy!


<u>Chicken Noodle Soup*</u>

   3 cups chicken broth

   1 chicken breast, diced

   2 Tablespoons avocado oil

   1 organic stalk of celery, chopped

   1 green onion, chopped

   1/4 cup cilantro, finely chopped

   1 zucchini, peeled, deseeded and created into zucchini noodles.

Himalayan sea Salt to taste

   Heat in a stock pot the oil and add the diced uncooked chicken breast. Allow to cook until no longer pink and the juices run clear.

Add the broth, celery and onions. Allow them to simmer until vegetables are tender. Next add the cilantro and zucchini noodles. Cook for 10 more minutes and season with salt to taste.

## Cabbage-Chicken Soup*

2 tbsp. coconut oil, Almond oil or Extra Virgin Olive Oil

1/2 of a small cabbage, cored and sliced thinly

3 stalks of organic celery, chopped

1/2 tsp. Himalayan sea salt

2 cloves of garlic, minced

1/2-1 tsp grated fresh ginger

2 and 1/2 cups of bone broth, chicken broth or vegetable broth

1 cup chopped or shredded leftover chicken (or any meat that you like)

Himalayan sea salt to taste

Fresh cilantro for garnish

Sauté the cabbage, and celery over medium high heat for 3-4 minutes, until veggies are tender, stirring often. Next add garlic and ginger and cook for another minute. Add the broth and cooked chicken to pot. Allow to simmer for 30 minutes. Garnish with fresh cilantro.


## Cabbage-Sauerkraut Soup*

8 oz. salt pork, rinsed and patted dry, then sliced into wide strips about 1/4" thick

2 tbsp. coconut oil, Almond oil or Extra Virgin Olive Oil

1 large head green cabbage, cored and thinly sliced

2 lb. organic sauerkraut, rinsed

4 cups of bone broth, chicken broth or vegetable broth

Himalayan sea salt to taste

In a medium size stock pot sauté pork strips on both sides for 5 minutes until the meat begins to brown. Next add the cabbage, sauerkraut, and broth of your choice. Bring the mixture to a boil, then reduce to a simmer and allow it to simmer for about 45 minutes, stirring occasionally. Once the dish is done you can pull the pork out and chop into bite size pieces and add it back to the pot.

## Pork and Cabbage Stew*

2 tbsp. coconut oil, Almond oil or Extra Virgin Olive Oil

1 lb. pork boneless shoulder, butt, or loin, cubed

3 cups of cold water

1 head green cabbage, cored and thinly sliced

1 onion or leek, diced

½ inch of fresh ginger, peeled and diced into large slices

1 Tablespoon organic apple cider vinegar

Himalayan Sea Salt to taste

In a medium size stock pot sauté the pork on both sides for 5 minutes until the meat begins to brown. Next add the rest of the ingredients to the stock pot. Bring the mixture to a boil, then reduce to a simmer and allow it to simmer for about 2 hours, stirring occasionally. Keep an eye on it you might need to add more water.


## Slower Cooker Bacon Cabbage Chuck Roast Stew*

½ pound of organic uncured nitrate free bacon, roughly diced

2 to 3 lbs. grass-fed chuck roast, cut in 2" pieces

2 large organic red onions, peeled and cut in slices

1 clove organic garlic, peeled and minced

1 head green cabbage, cored and thinly sliced

Himalayan sea salt to taste

1 sprig fresh organic thyme

2 cups of homemade beef bone broth

Himalayan sea salt to taste

Layer your slow cooker as follows: Bacon, onion, garlic, chuck roast, cabbage, thyme and then the broth.  Season with salt to taste. Cook on low for 7 hours. Ladle in bowls.


## Turmeric Chicken Soup*

5 cups chicken bone broth

2 tbsp. coconut oil, avocado oil or extra virgin olive oil

4 organic chicken breasts, cooked and shredded

2 cups cauliflower, diced into bite size pieces

1 medium onion, peeled and diced

3 celery stalks, diced

2 tsp ground turmeric

1 tsp ground ginger

Himalayan Sea salt to taste

2 springs of fresh parsley

In a medium size stock pot, add the oil and the onions until soft. Next add in the broth, turmeric, ginger, and salt, chicken along with the spring of parsley. Simmer on medium heat for 20-25 minutes or until the cauliflower has softened to your liking. Ladle into bowls.


## Broccoli and Bacon Soup*

1 lb. of nitrate-free uncured bacon, uncooked and roughly diced

1 medium onion, peeled and diced

1 large parsnip, peeled and diced

2 celery stalks, chopped

2 cloves of garlic, peeled and minced

6 cups bone broth, chicken broth or vegetable broth

1.5 pounds fresh broccoli, chopped

Himalayan sea salt to taste

In a stock pot over medium heat cook the bacon till almost done then add the onions, garlic, and celery. Cook for an additional 3 minutes, stirring the mixture. Don't burn the bacon. Add the rest of the ingredients to the pot and allow it simmer for 30 minutes.

Using an immersion blender, blend soup until smooth.  If you do not have an immersion blender, transfer soup in batches and blend until smooth. Ladle into bowls.

# Salads, Dressings and More

 A nutritionally dense diet doesn't have to be a full-time job. I am sure there are a hundred and one different variations on how to make a keto AIP salad. It all boils down to your food code, your taste buds and this is your journey. This is all about you. Use the list that I have given you and create some wonderful salads that you will love to eat. Twice a week I create a basic salad to store in my fridge that is made up of organic lettuce, red onions and deseeded cucumbers. I add whatever I feel that I am in the mood to eat to that basic salad or I just eat that basic salad along with some homemade dressing.

A healthy Keto AIP salads are made with leafy greens and Low GI non-starchy vegetables that are excellent for fast lunches and busy days.

Many over the counter salad dressings are filled with Trans fats, sugar, preservatives and artificial ingredients. You can easily make your salad dressings in a few moments. All the vinaigrette recipes can be prepared ahead and refrigerated in a mason jar with a tightly sealed lid up to 1 week.

Try to purchase vinegars that have no added sugar, or a malt vinegar, which generally contains gluten. It's super easy to read the label, my friends.

## Basic Vinaigrette*

1 cup of olive oil

$\frac{1}{4}$ cup of organic apple cider vinegar

1 teaspoon of garlic powder

1 teaspoon of onion powder

1 teaspoon of Himalayan sea salt

Pour all the ingredients in a mason jar with a lid and give a good shake to combine. Store in the refrigerator.


<u>Cucumber coconut milk ranch dressing *</u>

1 can of full fat coconut milk or coconut cream, refrigerate overnight

1 medium cucumber, peeled, seeds removed, grated on a large holes of a box grater.

2 tablespoons of minced shallots

1 garlic clove, minced

2 tablespoons of organic apple cider vinegar

1.5 tablespoons of fresh parsley, basil and dill chopped very finely

Himalayan sea salt to taste

Open the can of full-fat coconut milk after it has been refrigerated all night; scoop the cream off the top of the can and add it to a large mason jar, leaving the coconut water within the can.

Add 4 tablespoons of the coconut water into the coconut cream and whisk until smooth ( save some of the leftover coconut water; you may need to wish in an extra tablespoon or two after refrigerating your dressing, depending on  your desired thickness)

Add in the rest of the ingredients, close the lid tightly, shake until combined and refrigerate dressing for at least 30 minutes to let the flavors combine together. Store in the refrigerator.


## Cilantro Lime Dressing*

1 bunch of cilantro

Zest from 1 lime

Juice from 1 lime

1/4 - 1/2 tsp sea salt (to taste)

1/2 cup avocado oil

1/2 cup full fat coconut milk

Place all the ingredients into your food processor or blender and blend until smooth.

## Creamy Cilantro Avocado Dressing*

1 avocado, cut in half, deseeded and flash diced

3 TBSP avocado oil

Juice of 1 lime

Handful of cilantro leaves

1/4 Himalayan sea salt

Place everything in a blender and blend well.

## Avocado Bacon Broccoli Salad*

1 head of broccoli, cored removed and finely chopped

3 stalks of celery, chopped

4 slices of nitrate free and uncured bacon, cooked and crumbled

1/4 red onion, peeled and diced

1 large avocado, cut in half, deseeded and flesh diced

1 tbsp. apple cider vinegar

Himalayan sea salt to taste

Place everything in a large bowl and mix well. Season with sea salt to taste.


## Chicken Avocado Salad with Cilantro and Lime*

One rotisserie chicken, chopped

Two avocados, cut in half, deseeded and flesh diced

½ cup of green cabbage, shredded

5 green onions (scallions), white and pale green parts, minced

Juice of 2 limes

Two handfuls of fresh cilantro, chopped

Himalayan sea Salt to taste

One large Cucumber, peeled and deseeded

Place all the ingredients in a large bowl and squeeze the lime over it.


## Sardines Salad*

1 can sardines in olive oil or brine, drained

(I like the Wild Planet Wild Sardines brand)

1/4 lb. salad greens mix or spinach

2 sliced of nitrate free uncured bacon, cooked crispy and crumbled

1 Tablespoon olive oil

1 Tablespoon lemon juice

Himalayan sea salt to taste

Place the salad greens in a bowl and toss them the lemon juice and olive oil. Add the crumbled bacon and sardines. Season with sea salt to taste.

## Steak Salad*

6 oz. grass fed steak, cooked to your liking and cut into strips

2 cups of mixed greens or spinach

1 Tablespoon olive oil

1 Tablespoon lemon juice

 Himalayan sea salt to taste

Place the salad greens in a bowl and toss them the lemon juice and olive oil. Add the cooked steak. Season with sea salt to taste.

## Salmon Salad*

   1 avocado, cut in half, deseeded and flash diced

   2 cans of wild salmon, drained, bones and skin picked out/off

½ cup red onion, peeled and diced

2 cups of mixed greens or spinach

⅓ Cup olives of your choice (Kalamata, green or black)

2.5 oz. artichoke hearts, drained and diced

2 tbsp. lemon juice

1½ tsp dried dill

Himalayan sea salt to taste

Place everything in a large bowl and mix well. Season with sea salt to taste.


## Cucumber-Avocado Salad*

1 avocado, cut in half, deseeded and flesh diced

1 cucumber, peeled, deseeded and diced

1/4 red onion, peeled and diced

1/4 cup parsley or 1 Tsp dried

2 tsp. extra virgin olive oil, coconut oil, MCT oil or Avocado oil

Himalayan sea salt to taste

Place everything in a large bowl and mix well. Season with sea salt to taste.


## Avocado Cucumber Ginger blueberry Salad*

1 cucumber, peeled and diced small

1 avocado, cut in half, deseeded and flash diced

1 Tablespoon freshly ginger, peeled and minced

1 teaspoon lemon juice

1 Tablespoon extra-virgin olive oil, coconut oil, MCT oil or Avocado oil

¼ cup of blueberries

Himalayan sea salt to taste

Place everything in a large bowl and mix well. Season with sea salt to taste.

## House Rub*

　½ TBSP Himalayan Sea Salt

　2 TBSP Garlic Powder

　1 TBSP Dried Organic Oregano Leaf

　2 teaspoons of Dried Organic Thyme Leaf

　½ teaspoon of Organic Ground Ceylon Cinnamon

　1 teaspoon of Dried Shallots or Dried Minced Onion

　¼ teaspoon of Ground Ginger powder

　Place everything in a mason jar with a tightly sealed lid. Make sure to date & label.


## Grilled Guacamole Sliders*

　1 lb. ground organic turkey or grass-fed beef

　1 large avocado, cut in half, deseeded and flesh scooped out

　2 tbsp. fresh lime juice

1 tsp Himalayan sea salt

1/4 cup rough chopped cilantro

1 small onion, peeled and diced

Place in a medium size mixing bowl the avocado, cilantro, and onion. Mix well to combine. Next add your ground turkey or beef, lime juice, and sea salt, by hand mixing everything and form into patties. Cook until done. I cook mine about 5 minutes preside. Depending on how hot your grill is. I wrap my burgers in a large lettuce leaf as my bun.

## Keto AIP Slam Mushroom Burger*

8 large flat mushrooms (you want them as large as a burger)

1 tsp avocado oil

8 strips of nitrate free, uncured bacon, cooked

2lbs of ground organic turkey or grass-fed beef

1 organic red onion, peeled and cut into slices


## For the guacamole

1 avocado, cut in half, seed thrown away and flesh scooped out

Juice from half a lime

Himalayan sea salt to taste

Rinse off the mushrooms getting rid of any dirt or debris. Cut the stem off and put 2 stems aside. Brush both sides of the mushroom with the avocado oil. Place on the grill for 5 minutes on both sides.

In a bowl, mix the organic turkey or grass-fed beef with the onion. Diced up the stem from the mushroom 2 mushrooms and add that to the mixture.

In a bowl, make the guacamole and blend it well.

Grill the patty until done.

Layer the burger. Mushroom (you want the underside to be the inside of the bun), guacamole, bacon slice, red onion, patty and then top with another mushroom slice.


## Summer Squash Stir Fry*

2 TBS olive oil, avocado oil or coconut oil

1 lb. grass-fed ground beef or organic turkey

1 large zucchini, peeled, deseeded and diced

1 yellow squash - peeled, deseeded and diced

1 medium onion, peeled and diced

7-8 whole button mushrooms, rinsed and diced

$\frac{1}{2}$ tsp Himalayan sea salt

2 cloves of garlic, peeled and minced

1 tsp dried oregano

Over medium high heat add your oil and brown your meat. After it's almost done (not that much pink left). Add the rest of your ingredients. Cook until the vegetables are tender and enjoy!

Ground Beef Stroganoff*

    1 lb. grass fed ground beef

    1 medium onion, peeled and diced small

    1 clove garlic, peeled and minced

    8 oz. cremini or button mushrooms, rinsed and sliced

    1 cup chicken or beef broth

    2 tsp. coconut aminos

    1/3 cup cream from top of chilled can of coconut milk

    Juice from half a small lemon

    1/2 tsp. Himalayan sea salt or to taste

Over medium high heat brown the ground beef and add the onion to the pan to cook until tender. Add the salt to season. Next add the garlic and mushrooms to the pan. Stir to combine. Slowly add broth, stirring and using a wooden spoon scrape the bits off the bottom of the skillet. Lastly add coconut aminos. Allow this mixture to cook for additional 5 minutes. While this is cooking you want to gather 1/3 cup of coconut cream from the top of a chilled can of coconut milk. (You put the entire can in the fridge and allow it to get cold) Add the coconut/lemon juice mixture to the skillet right before serving. Give it a few stirs and make sure it is heated through and seasoned to your liking. Serve over rice cauliflower, zucchini noodles, or mashed cauliflower.

## Cinnamon burger sliders*

2 lbs. ground grass fed beef, organic ground turkey or organic ground chicken

2 tsp. cinnamon

1 tsp. Himalayan sea salt

Combine all the ingredients in a bowl and form into small patties. Cook on a hot grill until done and enjoy.

## Slow Cooker Cinnamon Chuck Roast and Onions*

4 lbs. chuck roast

2 onions, peeled and cut in half-moon slices

Ground Ceylon cinnamon

Garlic powder

Himalayan sea Salt

Place the onions in the bottom of slow cooker. Season the beef roast generously on all sides with salt, garlic powder, ground cinnamon. Lay roast on top of onions. Pour in water as required to submerge the roast halfway. Place cover on slow cooker. Set temperature to low and allow to cook for 8 hours


## Lemony Chicken or Turkey + Broccoli*

4 boneless, skinless Chicken Breasts or Turkey Breasts

1 large head broccoli, broken into florets

1 Tbsp. avocado, coconut or olive oil

Himalayan sea salt to taste

1 cup chicken stock, vegetable broth or bone broth

1/4 cup fresh squeezed lemon juice

3 cloves fresh garlic, minced or pressed

In a large skillet heat oil over medium-high heat. Season the chicken or turkey with the sea salt on both sides.

Cook chicken or turkey in the skillet for about 3-4 minutes per side or until golden brown. Remove and set aside. Add the garlic to sauté a few minutes. Next add in the broth and lemon juice to the skillet. Stir and scrape up the brown bits from the bottom of the pan. Lastly, place the broccoli in the pan and try to allow the broth to cover it. Simmer for about 10 minutes, until broccoli is bright green and tender-crisp and chicken or turkey is cooked through.

## Salmon Lime and roasted vegetables*

2 lbs. wild caught salmon filet

1 large zucchini, peeled, deseeded and cut into bite size pieces

1 bunch of asparagus, ends trimmed and cut into 3" pieces

1 red onion, peeled and cut into wedges

1.5 Tbsp. coconut, avocado oil, extra virgin olive oil, melted

2 fresh limes, juiced

2 fresh garlic cloves, peeled and minced

Himalayan sea salt to taste

Fresh parsley, or cilantro for garnish (optional)

Place parchment paper on a pan and heat the oven to 400 degrees f. Place the salmon filet skin side down, then arrange all the chopped veggies next to it. In a small bowl, whisk together melted coconut oil, lime juice and minced garlic. Drizzle over salmon and veggies to coat well. Toss veggies a bit. Season with sea salt.     Bake for 15-20 minutes in your preheated oven, or until salmon begins to flake.


## Bacon Burger Cabbage Stir Fry*

1 pound nitrate free uncured bacon, diced

1 pound ground grass fed beef

1 small onion, peeled and diced

3 cloves garlic, peeled and minced

1 small head of cabbage, cored and diced into small strips

1/2 teaspoon Himalayan sea salt or to taste

In a medium stock pot brown bacon and beef together until cooked.     Remove cooked meat and place in a bowl. Add the onion and garlic in the hot grease from the meat until onion has become softened. Next add the diced cabbage and stir fry until wilted. Add in the meat and season with salt to taste.


## Lemony Roast Chicken*

1 whole organic chicken

2 sprigs organic rosemary

2 tablespoons avocado oil

1 onion, peeled and cut into wedges

1 lemon, cut in wedges

2 garlic cloves, peeled

1 tablespoon Himalayan sea salt

Pre-heat oven to 350 degrees. Remove chicken from the packaging, and rinse well under cold water. Place chicken on a baking dish breast up. Make sure nothing is in the cavity and stuff the cavity with the rosemary, Lemon, onion and garlic cloves. Rub the entire chicken down with avocado oil. Season the chicken with the salt. Flip the chicken over, breast side down. Bake for about 1 hour and 30 minutes. All juice should run clear, make sure the chicken is done. The leg should easily fall apart form the body if pulled.


## Mushroom, Bacon, and Cauliflower Casserole*

1 lb. nitrate free uncured bacon, diced

1 onion, peeled and diced

1 tablespoon fresh thyme

6 garlic cloves, peeled and minced

1/2 teaspoon Himalayan sea salt

12 oz. sliced cremini mushrooms

4 oz. sliced shiitake mushrooms

1 head of cauliflower, diced very small

1/4 cup beef or chicken bone broth

1 cup fresh organic spinach

2 teaspoons coconut aminos

Preheat oven to 375 degrees F.

In a stock pot over medium heat cook the bacon pieces until crisp. Remove bacon from pot, reserving 1 tablespoon drippings in the pot. Set the bacon aside on a paper napkin. Add the onion, garlic, and thyme to the drippings. Cook for 3 minutes until slightly browned and tender. Add mushrooms and salt. Cook for 10 minutes, stirring occasionally. Stir in diced cauliflower and broth, cooking for 5 minutes. Add spinach, bacon, and coconut aminos, stirring until spinach has wilted. Place everything in a 2-quart baking dish. Bake for 25 minutes.

# Keto AIP Smoothies and Infused Waters

## Cucumber lemon Mint Infused Water*

4 sprigs of mint leaves

1 medium cucumber peeled, deseeded and sliced

2 lemon's washed, cut into quarters

2 quarts water

Place everything in a pitcher and refrigerator for at least an hour and drink over ice.

## Zingy Salted Lime Soda*

1 lime, juiced

25 oz. bottle of mineral water, seltzer or tonic water

1/8 teaspoon Himalayan sea salt (or to taste)

Place everything in a pitcher and refrigerator for at least an hour and drink over ice.

## Rosemary Mint Soda*

25 oz. bottle of mineral water, seltzer or tonic water

4 sprigs rosemary

4 sprigs mint

1 lime cut into 4 wedges

Place everything in a pitcher and refrigerator for at least an hour and drink over ice.

## Cucumber Basil Ice Cubes*

1 cucumber peeled, deseeded and diced

5 small basil leaves

Juice from 1 whole lime

2 cups of cups of filtered water

Place everything into the blender and blend well. Strain the mixture through a mesh strainer and then pour mixture into ice cube trays or molds. Freeze the trays for 4-5 hours (or overnight) until solid. Add these ice cubes to your favorite beverage.


## Cold Brew Matcha Iced Tea with Lemon and Mint*

6 cups filtered water

6 good quality Matcha tea bags

1 lemon sliced into wedges

2 fresh mint sprigs

Place everything in a pitcher and refrigerator for at least an hour and drink over ice.

## Antioxidant Wellness Tea*

1 cup boiling water.

1 tsp. freshly squeezed lemon juice

1 small knob of ginger, peeled and left whole

1/2 tbsp. Organic Apple Cider Vinegar.

1/4 tsp ground turmeric

Add all the ingredients in a cup or mug. Stir to mix well. Allow to cool a bit and enjoy. Be mindful of the large piece of ginger in your drink. You don't want to end up choking on that.


## Blueberries-Hibiscus Iced Tea*

8 cups water

1½ tbsp. dried mint

1½ tbsp. dried hibiscus flowers or 4 hibiscus tea bags

1 lb. blueberries, hulled

¼ cup lemon juice

   Bring the water to a boil and combine the mint and hibiscus in a tea ball. If you are using the tea bags don't add them to the ball just place them in the water. Once it boils. Allow the tea ball too steep for 15 minutes. Remove the tea ball and discard its contents. Allow the tea to cool to room temperature where you can pour it in a pitcher and place it in the fridge to chill for at least 30 minutes. I enjoy my tea warm therefore I heat it up in a cup before drinking. You may like it over ice in a glass after it has chilled in the fridge.


## "Bulletproof" Style Dandelion/Chicory Coffee*

   1 teaspoon roasted dandelion root

   1 teaspoon roasted chicory root

   16 ounces boiling water

   1 tablespoon MCT oil

   1 tablespoon coconut oil

Place the dandelion and chicory root in a tea ball. Bring the water to a boil.  Once it boils. Allow the tea ball too steep for 15 minutes. Remove the tea ball and discard its contents. Place the MCT oil, coconut oil, and "coffee" into a blender, making sure to lid tightly and place a kitchen towel over top to protect your hand. Blend for 30 seconds on high, until creamy and frothy. If this is your 1st time doing this it may be too much "oil" for you so you can cut the amount of "oil" in half.

## Cucumber Celery Lime Smoothie*

4 stalks of celery heart, chopped into large chunks

1 small cucumber, peeled, chopped, and the seeds removed

Juice from 1 lime

2 cups of water

1/2 cup ice

Place everything into a good blender and blend well.


## Berry Lemon ACV Drink*

2 tablespoons fresh or frozen blueberries

1 tablespoon organic apple cider vinegar

1 tablespoon lemon juice

Place everything in a pitcher and refrigerator for at least an hour and drink over ice.

# Smoothies

Remember this is your journey. Smoothies are a fantastic ways to get in a large amount of nutrients without having to actually chew!

You should always start with a healthy fatty base like full-fat canned coconut milk, MCT oil, avocado, coconut yogurt, coconut oil, flax seed oil or anything that is listed on our approved list of healthy fats. Next pick a low GI non starchy veggie from the approved list like cucumber, broccoli, spinach, celery, kale are all good examples.

You can even add in a ½ cup of organic blueberries or just skip this berry all together.

Don't forget to add some flavor boosters likes cinnamon, mint and ginger. We have a whole list of approved herbs and spices that you can choose from. Even add some unsweetened coconut flakes, chia or flax seeds if that is what you like but remember if you add chia seeds make sure you allow your smoothie to sit for a few minutes or mix the chia seeds with equal's amounts of water to thicken into a gel. People have been known to get these seeds stuck in their throats when eaten dry.

Be creative with your smoothies. If they are too thick, add more liquid, if they are too thin for your liking add less liquid. Play with the ingredients. Make a smoothie that you know you're going to drink. Every single smoothie has celery in it. The reason why celery is in every smoothie is it has super health benefits that range from reducing inflammation, regulates the body's alkaline balance, aids digestion, reduces "bad" cholesterol, reduces bloating, helps to prevent ulcers, lowers blood pressure, amps up your sex life, cancer fighter, excellent source of antioxidants and beneficial enzymes, in addition to vitamins and minerals such as vitamin K, vitamin C, potassium, folate and vitamin B6. If you don't like celery then just omit it.

I also suggest that you want to use a low carb keto friendly protein powder-go with an all-natural vegan, gluten free, dairy free, lactose free, no fillers, no synthetic nutrients, no artificial flavors or sweeteners, no preservatives , no pea protein  and soy free protein mix. This is why I use FIT Raw Meal, Garden of life brand products. No they are not endorsing me to say this. I picked this brand up after a long research study on my part. I am sure there are other brands just as good as this brand but I prefer this brand.

Become mindful and read labels. You want to stay clear of hidden poisons that can be in your protein powders. Here are 3 to be on the lookout for to avoid.

## Soy Protein Isolate

Soy protein has been a main ingredient in many protein powders for a while. Soy has been found to be toxic to the digestive system and creates the following concerns:

Disrupts thyroid and endocrine function

Interferes with leptin sensitivity which can cause metabolic syndrome

Throws off estrogen and testosterone balance

Blocks the body's ability to access key minerals like iron, zinc, calcium, and magnesium

It is also estimated that soy is over 95% genetically modified, and one of the most pesticide ridden crops on the market.

This makes any non-organic soy protein (especially isolate) found in protein powders, indigestible and toxic to the human physiology.

## Whey Protein Isolate

Whey protein can be a quality protein. Not many on the market are good to digest. If whey came from conventionally raised cows that have been fed non-organic grains and genetically modified foods, and been injected with antibiotics and hormones, which makes it not a good quality source of protein. You also need to keep in mind that this form of whey in an isolate format is not properly absorbed by the body.

If you do choose a whey protein, it is important to see where the whey has come from. Make sure it is from grass fed cows. Which are nutritionally superior compared to grain fed, and they contain an impressive amino acid and immune-supportive nutrient profile.

## Rice Protein

Same as the source of the whey protein, the kicker is where it comes from. Even though rice protein can be an acceptable source of protein but many that are not.

Thanks to a report unveiled earlier in 2014 by Mike Adams, we have been able to discover that there are many rice protein powders on the market that have been heavily contaminated with tungsten, cadmium, and lead. The reason for this high level of contamination is due to sourcing rice from China, where air pollution can trump the "organic" label placed on many products, including rice.

<u>Blueberry Coconut Yogurt Smoothie*</u>

   1 cup of coconut yogurt

   3 organic celery stalks

   10 frozen or fresh blueberries

   1 cup full fat coconut milk, unsweetened coconut milk or water

   1 cup of ice

Add all ingredients to a high speed blender and mix on high until smooth.

## Berry Smoothie*

1/4 cup frozen blueberries

3 organic celery stalks

1/4-1/2 Avocado, cut in half, seed discarded and flesh scooped   out

½ cup spinach or 1/2 cup romaine

(If you have hypothyroidism use the romaine)

1 Tbsp. apple cider vinegar

2 tsp Ceylon cinnamon

2 Tbsp. collagen peptides

2 Tbsp. MCT oil, coconut oil or flaxseed oil

1 cup of coconut milk or unsweetened coconut milk or water

1 cup of ice

Add all ingredients to a high speed blender and mix on high until smooth.


## Green Smoothie*

1 cup of water, full fat coconut milk or unsweetened coconut milk

1 tbsp. MCT oil or coconut oil

½ tsp lemon zest

1 tablespoon lemon juice

1 tablespoon lime juice

1 handful of spinach (replace with romaine if you have hypothyroidism)

3 organic celery stalks

1 cup of ice

Add all ingredients to a high speed blender and mix on high until smooth.


## Pumpkin Smoothie*

¾ cup full-fat coconut milk, unsweetened coconut milk or water

3 organic celery stalks

3 tablespoons pumpkin puree

1 tablespoon MCT oil, coconut oil or flaxseed oil

1 teaspoon matcha tea

½ avocado, cut in half seed discarded and flesh scooped out

¼ teaspoon ground Ceylon cinnamon

1/8 teaspoon ground ginger

1 cup of ice

Add all ingredients to a high speed blender and mix on high until smooth.


## Collagen Smoothie*

1/2 medium avocado, cut in half seed discarded and flesh scooped out

3 organic celery stalks

2 scoops Collagen

1 tbsp. chia seeds, soaked in 3 tbsp. water for 15 minutes

1 tbsp. coconut butter

3/4 cup full fat coconut milk, unsweetened coconut milk or water

1 1/4 cup water

1 cup of ice cubes

Add all ingredients to blender and blend until well-combined.


## Blueberry Matcha Smoothie*

2 tbsp. collagen peptides

3 organic celery stalks

1 tablespoon MCT Oil, flax seed oil or organic coconut oil

1 tsp Matcha powder

1/4 cup full fat canned coconut milk

1/4 cup frozen wild blueberries

1 cup of ice

8 oz. of water

Add all ingredients to blender and blend until well-combined.


## Cucumber Celery Lime Smoothie*

3 organic celery stalks

1 small cucumber, peeled, chopped, and the seeds removed

Juice from 1/2 lime

8 oz. of water

1 cup of ice

Place everything into a good blender and blend well.

The best patient to be is a well informed and an educated patient.

(Recipes as in the measured list of ingredients) and very short directions on how to combine those ingredients are not protected under the various forms of copyright law. This is because they fall under the designation of being the steps in a procedure and they're explicitly excluded form copyright.

Countries which are signatories to either the Berne convention or the Buenos Aires convention use the same basic standard to determine what is and isn't copyrighted although there are small local variations.

However, the exclusion on procedures is not a local variation.

What can be copyrights are the more complex directions that usually accompany the list of ingredients in modern recipes. As long as you rewrite any directions to be in your own words you've followed the law. Cooking something from a recipe recorded by someone else and sell it is legal.)

Knowledge is power, educate yourself and find the answer to your health care needs. Wisdom is a wonderful thing to seek. I hope this book will teach and encourage you to take leaps in your life to educate yourself for a happier & healthier life. You have to take ownership of your health.

Prayer for today:

Lord, please help me to get out of my own way so I don't miss out on the wonderful things you have for me. Help me to remember that your promises are true and you have always and will always provide my every need. Your word says, that you will bless me, exceedingly, abundantly and above all that I can ask or think. I want change, I want to be healthy and I want to learn how to heal my body. I step out on faith and I know you will guide me as I search for the truth.  I thank you for wisdom and spiritual guidance.

In Jesus' name I pray, Amen!

REFERENCES————

J. Karovičová, Milan Drdák, Gabriel Greif, & Hybenová E (1999). The choice of strains of Lactobacillus species for the lactic acid fermentation of vegetable juices. European Food Research and Technology 210(1):53-56. DOI: 10.1007/s002170050532

Quigley L, et al. (2011). Molecular approaches to analysing the microbial composition of raw milk and raw milk cheese. International Journal of Food Microbiology 150(2-3):81-94. PMID 21868118

Donovan SM & Shamir R (2014). Introduction to the yogurt in nutrition initiative and the First Global Summit on the health effects of yogurt. The American Journal of Clinical Nutrition 99(5 Suppl):1209S-1211S. PMID 24646825

Beermann C & Hartung J (2013). Physiological properties of milk ingredients released by fermentation. Food & Function 4(2):185-199. PMID 23111492

Hennessy AA, et al. (2012). The production of conjugated alpha-linolenic, gamma-linolenic and stearidonic acids by strains of bifidobacteria and propionibacteria. Lipids 47(3):313-327. PMID 22160449

Parvez S, Malik KA, Ah Kang S, & Kim HY (2006). Probiotics and their fermented food products are beneficial for health. Journal of Applied Microbiology 100(6):1171-1185. PMID 16696665

Padilla B, et al. (2012). Evaluation of oligosaccharide synthesis from lactose and lactulose using beta-galactosidases from Kluyveromyces isolated from artisanal cheeses. Journal of Agricultural and Food Chemistry 60(20):5134-5141. PMID 22559148

USDA ARS (2013). USDA national nutrient database for standard reference, release 26. Nutrient Data Laboratory homepage.

Wang H, Livingston KA, Fox CS, Meigs JB, & Jacques PF (2013). Yogurt consumption is associated with better diet quality and metabolic profile in American men and women. Nutrition Research 33(1):18-26. PMID 23351406

Adolfsson O, Meydani SN, & Russel RM (2004). Yogurt and gut function. The American Journal of Clinical Nutrition 80:245-256. PMID 15277142

Keszei AP, Schouten LJ, Goldbohm RA, & van den Brandt PA (2010). Dairy intake and the risk of bladder cancer in the Netherlands Cohort Study on Diet and Cancer. American Journal of Epidemiology 171(4):436-446. PMID 20042437

Sonestedt E, et al. (2011). Dairy products and its association with incidence of cardiovascular disease: the Malmo diet and cancer cohort. European journal of epidemiology 26(8):609-618. PMID 21660519

Adegboye AR, et al. (2012). Intake of dairy products in relation to periodontitis in older Danish adults. Nutrients 4(9):1219-1229. PMID 23112910

Siddappa V, Nanjegowda DK, & Viswanath P (2012). Occurrence of aflatoxin M(1) in some samples of UHT, raw & pasteurized milk from Indian states of Karnataka and Tamilnadu. Food and Chemical Toxicology 50(11):4158-4162. PMID 22939935

Prandini A, et al. (2009). On the occurrence of aflatoxin M1 in milk and dairy products. Food and Chemical Toxicology 47(5):984-991. PMID 18037552

Linares DM, Martin MC, Ladero V, Alvarez MA, & Fernandez M (2011). Biogenic amines in dairy products. Critical Reviews in Food Science and Nutrition 51(7):691-703. PMID 21793728

Redruello B, et al. (2013). A fast, reliable, ultra high performance liquid chromatography method for the simultaneous determination of amino acids, biogenic amines and ammonium ions in cheese, using diethyl ethoxymethylenemalonate as a derivatising agent. Food Chemistry 139(1-4):1029-1035. PMID 23561206

Buckenhuskes HJ (1997). Fermented vegetables. Food Microbiology: Fundamentals and Frontiers, eds Doyle PD, Beuchat LR, & Montville TJ (ASM Press, Washington, DC), 2nd Ed, pp 595-609. ISBN 9781555811174

Bering S, et al. (2006). A lactic acid-fermented oat gruel increases non-haem iron absorption from a phytate-rich meal in healthy women of childbearing age. The British Journal of Nutrition 96(1):80-85. PMID 16869994

Proulx AK & Reddy MB (2007). Fermentation and lactic acid addition enhance iron bioavailability of maize. Journal of Agricultural and Food Chemistry 55(7):2749-2754. PMID 17355139

Scheers N, Rossander-Hulthen L, Torsdottir I, & Sandberg AS (2015). Increased iron bioavailability from lactic-fermented vegetables is likely an effect of promoting the formation of ferric iron (Fe). European Journal of Nutrition. PMID 25672527

Flint HJ (2012). The impact of nutrition on the human microbiome. Nutrition Reviews 70 Suppl 1:S10-13. PMID 22861801

Scott KP, Gratz SW, Sheridan PO, Flint HJ, & Duncan SH (2013). The influence of diet on the gut microbiota. Pharmacological Research: The Official Journal of the Italian Pharmacological Society 69(1):52-60. PMID 23147033

FAO/WHO (2001). Report on Joint FAO/WHO Expert Consultation on Evaluation of Health and Nutritional Properties of Probiotics in Food Including Powder Milk with Live Lactic Acid Bacteria.

Jalanka-Tuovinen J, et al. (2011). Intestinal microbiota in healthy adults: temporal analysis reveals individual and common core and relation to intestinal symptoms. PloS One 6(7):e23035. PMID 21829582

Reuter G (2001). The Lactobacillus and Bifidobacterium microflora of the human intestine:

composition and succession. Current Issues in Intestinal Microbiology 2(2):43-53. PMID 11721280

Turroni F, et al. (2014). Molecular dialogue between the human gut microbiota and the host: a Lactobacillus and Bifidobacterium perspective. Cellular and Molecular Life Sciences: CMLS 71(2):183-203. PMID 23516017

Veiga P, et al. (2014). Changes of the human gut microbiome induced by a fermented milk product. Scientific Reports 4:6328. PMID 25209713

Round JL & Mazmanian SK (2009). The gut microbiota shapes intestinal immune responses during health and disease. Nature Reviews. Immunology 9(5):313-323. PMID 19343057

Champagne CP, Ross RP, Saarela M, Hansen KF, & Charalampopoulos D (2011). Recommendations for the viability assessment of probiotics as concentrated cultures and in food matrices. International Journal of Food Microbiology 149(3):185-193. PMID 21803436

Derrien M & van Hylckama Vlieg JE (2015). Fate, activity, and impact of ingested bacteria within the human gut microbiota. Trends in Microbiology 23(6):354-366. PMID 25840765

Lee YK, et al. (2000). Quantitative approach in the study of adhesion of lactic acid bacteria to intestinal cells and their competition with enterobacteria. Applied and Environmental Microbiology 66(9):3692-3697. PMID 10966378

Ouwehand AC, Tuomola EM, Lee YK, & Salminen S (2001). Microbial interactions to intestinal mucosal models. Methods in Enzymology 337:200-212. PMID 11398429

van Bokhorst-van de Veen H, et al. (2012). Modulation of Lactobacillus plantarum gastrointestinal robustness by fermentation conditions enables identification of bacterial robustness markers. PloS One 7(7):e39053. PMID 22802934

Marteau P, Minekus M, Havenaar R, & Huis in't Veld JH (1997). Survival of lactic acid bacteria in a dynamic model of the stomach and small intestine: validation and the effects of bile. Journal of Dairy Science 80(6):1031-1037. PMID 9201571

van Bokhorst-van de Veen H, van Swam I, Wels M, Bron PA, & Kleerebezem M (2012). Congruent strain specific intestinal persistence of Lactobacillus plantarum in an intestine-mimicking in vitro system and in human volunteers. PloS One 7(9):e44588. PMID 22970257

Uyeno Y, Sekiguchi Y, & Kamagata Y (2008). Impact of consumption of probiotic lactobacilli-containing yogurt on microbial composition in human feces. International Journal of Food Microbiology 122(1-2):16-22. PMID 18077045

Saxelin M, et al. (2010). Persistence of probiotic strains in the gastrointestinal tract when administered as capsules, yoghurt, or cheese. International Journal of Food Microbiology 144(2):293-300. PMID 21074284

Lim SM & Im DS (2009). Screening and characterization of probiotic lactic acid bacteria isolated from Korean fermented foods. Journal of Microbiology and Biotechnology 19(2):178-186. PMID 19307768

Lee KE, Choi UH, & Ji GE (1996). Effect of kimchi in intake on the composition of human large intestinal bacteria. Korean J Food Sci Technol 28:981-986. Abstract

Vitetta L, Briskey D, Alford H, Hall S, & Coulson S (2014). Probiotics, prebiotics and the gastrointestinal tract in health and disease. Inflammopharmacology 22(3):135-154. PMID 24633989

Kirjavainen PV, Arvola T, Salminen SJ, & Isolauri E (2002). Aberrant composition of gut microbiota of allergic infants: a target of bifidobacterial therapy at weaning? Gut 51(1):51-55. PMID 12077091

Hattori K, et al. (2003). [Effects of administration of bifidobacteria on fecal microflora and clinical symptoms in infants with atopic dermatitis]. Arerugi = [Allergy] 52(1):20-30. PMID 12598719

Isolauri E, Arvola T, Sutas Y, Moilanen E, & Salminen S (2000). Probiotics in the management of atopic eczema. Clinical and Experimental Allergy: Journal of the British Society for Allergy and Clinical Immunology 30(11):1604-1610. PMID 11069570

Neish AS, et al. (2000). Prokaryotic regulation of epithelial responses by inhibition of IkappaB-alpha ubiquitination. Science 289(5484):1560-1563. PMID 10968793

Schiffrin EJ, Brassart D, Servin AL, Rochat F, & Donnet-Hughes A (1997). Immune modulation of blood leukocytes in humans by lactic acid bacteria: criteria for strain selection. The American Journal of Clinical Nutrition 66(2):515S-520S. PMID 9250141

Lee YK & Puong KY (2002). Competition for adhesion between probiotics and human gastrointestinal pathogens in the presence of carbohydrate. The British Journal of Nutrition 88 Suppl 1:S101-108. PMID 12215184

Creagh EM & O'Neill LA (2006). TLRs, NLRs and RLRs: a trinity of pathogen sensors that co-operate in innate immunity. Trends in Immunology 27(8):352-357. PMID 16807108

Hughes DT & Sperandio V (2008). Inter-kingdom signalling: communication between bacteria and their hosts. Nature Reviews. Microbiology 6(2):111-120. PMID 18197168

Botic T, Klingberg TD, Weingartl H, & Cencic A (2007). A novel eukaryotic cell culture model to study antiviral activity of potential probiotic bacteria. International Journal of Food Microbiology 115(2):227-234. PMID 17261339

Juntunen M, Kirjavainen PV, Ouwehand AC, Salminen SJ, & Isolauri E (2001). Adherence of probiotic bacteria to human intestinal mucus in healthy infants and during rotavirus infection. Clinical and Diagnostic Laboratory Immunology 8(2):293-296. PMID 11238211

Resta-Lenert S & Barrett KE (2003). Live probiotics protect intestinal epithelial cells from the effects of infection with enteroinvasive Escherichia coli (EIEC). Gut 52(7):988-997. PMID 12801956

Banasaz M, Norin E, Holma R, & Midtvedt T (2002). Increased enterocyte production in gnotobiotic rats mono-associated with Lactobacillus rhamnosus GG. Applied and Environmental Microbiology 68(6):3031-3034. PMID 12039764

Deplancke B & Gaskins HR (2001). Microbial modulation of innate defense: goblet cells and the intestinal mucus layer. The American Journal of Clinical Nutrition 73(6):1131S-1141S. PMID 11393191

Otte JM & Podolsky DK (2004). Functional modulation of enterocytes by gram-positive and gram-negative microorganisms. American Journal of Physiology. Gastrointestinal and Liver Physiology 286(4):G613-626. PMID 15010363

O'Shea EF, et al. (2009). Characterization of enterocin- and salivaricin-producing lactic acid bacteria from the mammalian gastrointestinal tract. FEMS Microbiology Letters 291(1):24-34. PMID 19076236

Pridmore RD, Pittet AC, Praplan F, & Cavadini C (2008). Hydrogen peroxide production by Lactobacillus johnsonii NCC 533 and its role in anti-Salmonella activity. FEMS Microbiology Letters 283(2):210-215. PMID 18435747

Heller L (2009). Danisco breaks down probiotics market. (Nutra Ingredients, USA).

Cook MT, Tzortzis G, Charalampopoulos D, & Khutoryanskiy VV (2012). Microencapsulation of probiotics for gastrointestinal delivery. Journal of Controlled Release: Official Journal of the Controlled Release Society 162(1):56-67. PMID 22698940

Starling S (2009). Probiotics must meet Europe's new health claim laws head on.

Oliveira RP, et al. (2009). Effect of different prebiotics on the fermentation kinetics, probiotic survival and fatty acids profiles in nonfat symbiotic fermented milk. International Journal of Food Microbiology 128(3):467-472. PMID 19000641

Reid G (2008). How science will help shape future clinical applications of probiotics. Clinical Infectious Diseases: An Official Publication of the Infectious Diseases Society of America 46 Suppl 2:S62-66; discussion S144-151. PMID 18181725

Govender M, et al. (2014). A review of the advancements in probiotic delivery: Conventional vs. non-conventional formulations for intestinal flora supplementation. AAPS PharmSciTech 15(1):29-43. PMID 24222267

Herbel SR, et al. (2013). Species-specific quantification of probiotic lactobacilli in yoghurt by quantitative real-time PCR. Journal of Applied Microbiology 115(6):1402-1410. PMID 24024971

Dunlap BS, Yu H, & Elitsur Y (2009). The probiotic content of commercial yogurts in West Virginia. Clinical Pediatrics 48(5):522-527. PMID 19246412

Park KY, Jeong JK, Lee YE, & Daily JW, 3rd (2014). Health benefits of kimchi (Korean fermented vegetables) as a probiotic food. Journal of Medicinal Food 17(1):6-20. PMID 24456350

Lee D, Kim S, Cho J, & Kim J (2008). Microbial population dynamics and temperature changes during fermentation of kimjang kimchi. Journal of Microbiology 46(5):590-593. PMID 18974963

Lee JS, et al. (2005). Analysis of kimchi microflora using denaturing gradient gel electrophoresis. International Journal of Food Microbiology 102(2):143-150. PMID 15992614

Kim M & Chun J (2005). Bacterial community structure in kimchi, a Korean fermented vegetable food, as revealed by 16S rRNA gene analysis. International Journal of Food Microbiology 103(1):91-96. PMID 16084269

Lee J, Hwang KT, Heo MS, Lee JH, & Park KY (2005). Resistance of Lactobacillus plantarum KCTC 3099 from Kimchi to oxidative stress. Journal of Medicinal Food 8(3):299-304. PMID 16176138

Lee JH, Kweon DH, & Lee SC (2006). Isolation and characterization of an immunopotentiating factor from Lactobacillus plantarum in kimchi: assessment of immunostimulatory activities. . Food Sci Biotechnol 15:877-883. Abstract

Hur HJ, Lee KW, & Lee HJ (2004). Production of nitric oxide, tumor necrosis factor-alpha and interleukin-6 by RAW264.7 macrophage cells treated with lactic acid bacteria isolated from kimchi. BioFactors 21(1-4):123-125. PMID 15630182

Jang SE, et al. (2013). Lactobacillus plantarum HY7712 ameliorates cyclophosphamide-induced immunosuppression in mice. Journal of microbiology and biotechnology 23(3):414-421. PMID 23462016

Chae OW, Shin KS, Chung H, & Choe TB (1998). Immunostimulation effects of mice fed with cell lysate of Lactobacillus plantarum isolated from kimchi. Korean J Biotech Bioeng 13:424-430. Article

Kim NH, et al. (2008). Lipid profile lowering effect of Soypro fermented with lactic acid bacteria isolated from Kimchi in high-fat diet-induced obese rats. BioFactors 33(1):49-60. PMID 19276536

Kwon JY, Cheigh HS, & Song YO (2004). Weight reduction and lipid lowering effects of kimchi lactic acid powder in rats fed high fat diets. Korean J Food Sci Technol 36:1014-1019. Article

Ahn DK, Han TW, Shin HY, Jin IN, & Ghim SY (2003). Diversity and antibacterial activity of lactic acid bacteria isolated from kimchi. Korean J Microbiol Biotechnol 31:191-196. Abstract

Tang, M., Ponsonby, A-L., Orsini, F., Tey, D., Robinson, M., Su, E. L., Licciardi, P., Burks, W., and Donath, S., (2015). Administration of a probiotic with peanut oral immunotherapy: A randomized trial. The Journal of Allergy and Clinical Immunology. 135 (3): 737-44.PMID 25592987

Battcock, M & Azam-Ali, S 1998, 'Fermented fruits and vegetables: A global perspective', FAO Agricultural Services Bulletin, no. 134, viewed 18 July 2016, <http://www.fao.org/docrep/x0560e/x0560e00.htm#con&gt;

Kechagia, M Basoulis, D SKonstantopoulou, S Dimitriadi, D Gyftopoulou, K Skarmoutsou, K and Fakiri, EM 2013, Health Benefits of Probiotics: A Review, ISRN Nutrition, vol. 2013, Article ID 481651

Tillisch K, Labus J, Kilpatrick L, Jiang Z, Stains J, Ebrat B, Guyonnet D, Legrain-Raspaud S, Trotin B, Naliboff B, & Mayer EA 2013, Consumption of fermented milk product with probiotic modulates brain activity, Gastroenterology, no. 144, no. 7, pp. 1394-1401

Selhub, EM, Logan, AC, & Bested, AC 2014, 'Fermented foods, microbiota, and mental health: ancient practice meets nutritional psychiatry', Journal of Physiological Anthropology.

Derrien M & van Hylckama Vlieg JE 2015, 'Fate, activity, and impact of ingested bacteria within the human gut microbiota', Trends in Microbiology,23, no. 6, pp354-366.

den Besten, G, van Eunen, K, Groen, AK, Venema, K, Reijngoud, D, & Bakker, BM 2013, 'The role of short-chain fatty acids in the interplay between diet, gut microbiota, and host energy metabolism', Journal Of Lipid Research, vol. 54, no. 9, pp. 2325-2340.Farnworth ER (2008). Handbook of Fermented Functional Foods (CRC Press, Boca Raton, FL, USA). ISBN 9781420053265

Rolle R & Satin M (2002). Basic requirements for the transfer of fermentation technologies to developing countries. International Journal of Food Microbiology 75(3):181-187. PMID

http://www.westonaprice.org/health-topics/lacto-fermentation/

http://bodyecology.com/articles/boost_thyroid_energy.php

http://www.startribune.com/pizza-still-counts-as-a-veggie/134208058/

http://thenewpyramid.blogspot.com/2014/03/the-food-pyramid-is-lie-part-1-history.html

https://www.annalect.com/the-evolution-of-advertising-in-the-food-and-beverage-industry/

https://en.wikipedia.org/wiki/Food_marketing

https://en.wikipedia.org/wiki/History_of_marketing

https://www.tesh.com/articles/the-food-we-eat-today-is-higher-in-calories-and-lower-in-nutrients/

https://en.wikipedia.org/wiki/History_of_bread

https://superhumancoach.com/negative-effects-of-non-organic-un-rinsed-vegetables/

https://priceonomics.com/the-food-industrial-complex/

Alqasoumi, S., Al-Sohaibani, M., Al-Howiriny, T., Al-Yahya, M., & Rafatullah, S. (2009). Rocket "Eruca sativa": A salad herb with potential gastric anti-ulcer activity. World Journal of Gastroenterology : WJG, 15(16), 1958–1965. http://doi.org/10.3748/wjg.15.1958

Boyer, J., & Liu, R. H. (2004). Apple phytochemicals and their health benefits. Nutrition Journal, 3(5). http://doi.org/10.1186/1475-2891-3-5

Chandrashekhar, V. M., et al. (2011). "Anti-allergic activity of German chamomile (Matricaria recutita L.) in mast cell mediated allergy model." Journal of ethnopharmacology 137(1), 336-340. Retrieved from:

https://www.sciencedirect.com/science/article/pii/S0
378874111003941

Chen, Bing-Hung, et al. (2009). "Antiallergic
potential on RBL-2H3 cells of some phenolic
constituents of Zingiber Officinale (Ginger)." Journal
of Natural Products 72(5), 950-953. Retrieved
from:
https://pubs.acs.org/doi/abs/10.1021/np800555y

Kaiser, M.S. Youssouf, S.A. Tasduq, S. Singh, S.C.
Sharma, G.D. Singh, V.K. Gupta, B.D. Gupta, and
R.K. Johri, Anti-Allergic Effects of Herbal Product
from Allium Cepa (Bulb), Journal of Medicinal Food.
April 2009, 12(2): 374-382. Retrieved from:
https://www.liebertpub.com/doi/abs/10.1089/jmf.20
07.0642

Negro. D. et al. (2012). "Polyphenol compounds in
artichoke plant tissues and varieties." Journal of
Food Science. 77(2):C244-252. Retrieved from:
https://www.ncbi.nlm.nih.gov/pubmed/22251096

Siddaraju, M. N., Dharmesh, S. M. (2007).
"Inhibition of gastric H+, K+-ATPase and
Helicobacter pylori growth by phenolic antioxidants
of Zingiber officinale." Mol Nutr Food Res. 2007
Mar;51(3):324-32. Retrieved from:
http://www.ncbi.nlm.nih.gov/pubmed/17295419

Theoharides, T. C. (2009). "Luteolin as a therapeutic option for multiple sclerosis." Journal of Neuroinflammation, 6(29). http://doi.org/10.1186/1742-2094-6-29

Tomomasa KANDA, Hiroshi AKIYAMA, Akio YANAGIDA, Masayuki TANABE, Yukihiro GODA, Masatake TOYODA, Reiko TESHIMA & Yukio SAITO (2014) Inhibitory Effects of Apple Polyphenol on Induced Histamine Release from RBL-2H3 Cells and Rat Mast Cells, Bioscience, Biotechnology, and Biochemistry, 62:7, 1284-1289, DOI: 10.1271/bbb.62.1284

Zarfeshany, A., Asgary, S., & Javanmard, S. H. (2014). Potent health effects of pomegranate. Advanced Biomedical Research, 3, 100. http://doi.org/10.4103/2277-9175.129371

de Onis M, Monteiro C, Akre J, Glugston G. The worldwide magnitude of protein-energy malnutrition: an overview from the WHO Global Database on Child Growth. Bull World Health Organ. 1993;71:703-12. PMID: 8313488

Yoshida H, Tsuji K, Sakata T, Nakagawa A, Morita S. Clinical study of tongue pain. Serum zinc, vitamin B12, folic acid, and copper concentrations, and systemic disease. Br J Oral Maxillofac Surg. 2010;48:469-72. PMID: 19735964

Powers JM, Buchanan GR. Iron deficiency anemia in toddlers to teens: How to manage when prevention fails. Contemporary Pediatrics. 2014;31(5).

Williams ME. Examining the fingernails when evaluating presenting symptoms in elderly patients. Medscape. November 23, 2009. Available at: http://www.medscape.com/viewarticle/712251. Accessed May 24, 2017.

Bethel M, Carbone LD, Lohr KM, Machua W. Osteoporosis. Medscape Drugs & Diseases from WebMD. Updated: May 10, 2017. Available at: http://emedicine.medscape.com/article/330598-overview. Accessed May 24, 2017.

Tangpricha V, Khazai NB. Vitamin D deficiency and related disorders. Medscape Drugs & Diseases from WebMD. Updated: October 10, 2016. Available at: http://emedicine.medscape.com/article/128762-overview. Accessed May 24, 2017.

Lima GA, Paranhos Neto Fde P, Pereira GR, Gomes CP, Farias ML. Osteoporosis management in patient with renal function impairment. Arq Bras Endocrinol Metabol. 2014 Jul;58(5):530-9. PMID: 25166044

Schwarz SM, Greer FR, Finberg L. Rickets. Medscape Drugs & Diseases from WebMD. Updated: March 29, 2017. Available at: http://emedicine.medscape.com/article/985510-overview. Accessed May 24, 2017.

Canadian Paediatric Society. A risk of northern climate! Paediatr Child Health. 2002 Dec;7(10):680. PMID: 20046448

American Thyroid Association. Goiter. Available at: http://www.thyroid.org/goiter/. Accessed May 24, 2017.

Drutel A, Archambeaud F, Caron P. Selenium and the thyroid gland: more good news for clinicians. Clin Endocrinol (Oxf). 2013 Feb;78(2):155-64. PMID: 23046013

Ward BW, Schiller JS, Goodman RA. Multiple chronic conditions among US adults: a 2012 update. Prev Chronic Dis. 2014;11:E62.

Centers for Disease Control and Prevention. Leading causes of death and numbers of deaths, by sex, race, and Hispanic origin: United States, 1980 and 2014 (Table 19). Health, United States, 2015. https://www.cdc.gov/nchs/data/hus/hus15.pdf#019[PDF - 13.4 MB]. Accessed June 21, 2017.

Ogden CL, Carroll MD, Fryar CD, Flegal KM. Prevalence of obesity among adults and youth: United States, 2011-2014. NCHS Data Brief. 2015 Nov;(219):1-8.

Brault MW, Hootman J, Helmick CG, Theis KA, Armour BS. Prevalence and most common causes of disability among adults, United States, 2005. MMWR. 2009;58(16):421-426.

Barbour KE, Helmick CG, Boring M, Brady TJ. Prevalence of doctor-diagnosed arthritis and arthritis-attributable activity limitation—United States, 2013-2015. MMWR. 2017;66(9):246-253.

Centers for Disease Control and Prevention. National Diabetes Fact Sheet, 2011. http://www.cdc.gov/diabetes/pubs/pdf/ndfs_2011.pdf[PDF - 2.66 MB] Accessed December 20, 2013.

US Department of Health and Human Services. Healthy People 2020: Physical Activity. https://www.healthypeople.gov/2020/topics-objectives/topic/physical-activity/objectives. Accessed June 9, 2017.

Benjamin EJ, Blaha MJ, Chiuve SE, et al. Heart disease and stroke statistics—2017 update: a report from the American Heart Association. Circulation. 2017;135:e1-e458.

Jackson SL, Coleman King SM, Zhao L, Cogswell ME. Prevalence of sodium intake in the United States. 2016;64(52):1394–1397.

Centers for Disease Control and Prevention. Nutrition, Physical Activity, and Obesity: Data, Trends and Maps. https://www.cdc.gov/nccdphp/dnpao/data-trends-maps/index.html. Accessed June 7, 2017.

Jamal A, King BA, Neff LJ, Whitmill J, Babb SD, Graffunder CM. Current cigarette smoking among adults — United States, 2005–2015. 2016;65(44):1205–1211.

The Health Consequences of Smoking—50 Years of Progress: A Report of the Surgeon General. Atlanta, GA: US Dept. of Health and Human Services, Centers for Disease Control and Prevention; 2014. http://www.surgeongeneral.gov/library/reports/50-years-of-progress/full-report.pdf. Accessed February 7, 2014.

Centers for Disease Control and Prevention. Alcohol and Public Health: Alcohol Related Disease Impact (ARDI). www.cdc.gov/ardi. Accessed June 1, 2017.

Centers for Disease Control and Prevention. Binge Drinking. https://www.cdc.gov/alcohol/fact-sheets/binge-drinking.htm. Accessed June 1, 2017.

Kanny D, Liu Y, Brewer RD, Lu H. Binge Drinking — United States, 2011. 2013;62 (Suppl):77-80.

Esser MB, Hedden SL, Kanny D, Brewer RD, Gfroerer JC, Naimi TS. Prevalence of alcohol dependence among us adult drinkers, 2009-2011. Prev Chronic Dis. 2014;11:E206.

Gerteis J, Izrael D, Deitz D, LeRoy L, Ricciardi R, Miller T, Basu J. Multiple Chronic Conditions Chartbook.[PDF - 10.62 MB] AHRQ Publications No, Q14-0038. Rockville, MD: Agency for Healthcare Research and Quality; 2014. Accessed November 18, 2014.

Benjamin EJ, Blaha MJ, Chiuve SE, et al. Heart disease and stroke statistics—2017 update: a report from the American Heart Association. Circulation. 2017;135:e1-e458.

National Cancer Institute. Cancer Prevalence and Cost of Care Projections. http://costprojections.cancer.gov/. Accessed December 23, 2013.

American Diabetes Association. The Cost of Diabetes. http://www.diabetes.org/advocacy/news-events/cost-of-diabetes.html. Accessed December 23, 2013.

Centers for Disease Control and Prevention. Arthritis Cost Statistics. http://www.cdc.gov/arthritis/data_statistics/cost.htm. Accessed December 23, 2013.

Finkelstein EA, Trogdon JG, Cohen JW, Dietz W. Annual medical spending attributable to obesity: payer- and service-specific estimates. Health Aff. 2009;28(5):w822-31.

Sacks JJ, Gonzales KR, Bouchery EE, Tomedi LE, Brewer RD. 2010 National and State Costs of Excessive Alcohol Consumption. Am J Prev Med. 2015; 49(5):e73–e79.

http://www.healthtalk.org/peoples-experiences/long-term-conditions/living-multiple-health-problems/causes-health-problems-certain-and-uncertain

http://realfarmacy.com/cause-depression/

http://www.dnaindia.com/health/report-green-tea-helps-fight-autoimmune-disease-1550712

http://life.gaiam.com/article/liquid-healing-herbal-teas-fight-inflammation

http://umm.edu/health/medical/altmed/herb/eucalyptus

http://www.drweil.com/drw/u/QAA142972/Anti-Inflammatory-Herbs.com

https://www.ncbi.nlm.nih.gov/pubmed/25360509

http://sciencenetlinks.com/student-teacher-sheets/cells-your-body/

https://www.perfectketo.com/keto-healthy-ketosis-vs-ketoacidosis/

https://www.ncbi.nlm.nih.gov/pubmed/22673594

https://www.ncbi.nlm.nih.gov/pubmed/25402637

https://www.ncbi.nlm.nih.gov/pubmed/9832569

https://www.ncbi.nlm.nih.gov/pmc/articles/PMC2367001/

https://www.ncbi.nlm.nih.gov/pmc/articles/PMC2649682/

https://www.ncbi.nlm.nih.gov/pubmed/15123336

https://www.ncbi.nlm.nih.gov/pubmed/21130529

http://ethos.bl.uk/OrderDetails.do?uin=uk.bl.ethos.581361

http://time.com/4609015/ketogenic-diet-explained/

https://authoritynutrition.com/ketogenic-diet-101/

http://articles.mercola.com/ketogenic-diet.aspx

http://draxe.com/truth-about-the-controversial-ketogenic-diet/

http://www.phoenixhelix.com/2013/01/18/comparison-of-3-healing-diets/

http://autoimmunewellness.com/our-story/

http://empoweredsustenance.com/gaps-diet/

http://health.usnews.com/health-news/health-wellness/articles/2015/01/16/is-the-autoimmune-paleo-diet-legit

http://www.gapsdiet.com/gaps-outline.html

http://time.com/4609015/ketogenic-diet-explained/

https://authoritynutrition.com/ketogenic-diet-101/

http://articles.mercola.com/ketogenic-diet.aspx

http://draxe.com/truth-about-the-controversial-ketogenic-diet/

http://www.phoenixhelix.com/2013/01/18/comparison-of-3-healing-diets/

http://autoimmunewellness.com/our-story/

http://empoweredsustenance.com/gaps-diet/

http://health.usnews.com/health-news/health-wellness/articles/2015/01/16/is-the-autoimmune-paleo-diet-legit

http://www.gapsdiet.com/gaps-outline.html

1, 3 Mark's Daily Apple May 19, 2012

2 New York Times May 12, 2016

4 American College of Sports Medicine, 2012 World Congress on Exercise in Medicine

https://www.ncbi.nlm.nih.gov/pubmed/21949221

http://www.ncbi.nlm.nih.gov/pubmed/10885323

http://www.ncbi.nlm.nih.gov/pubmed/12841427

http://www.ncbi.nlm.nih.gov/pubmed/15113714

http://www.ncbi.nlm.nih.gov/pubmed/1314519

http://www.ncbi.nlm.nih.gov/pubmed/12936919

http://www.ncbi.nlm.nih.gov/pubmed/11090291

http://www.ncbi.nlm.nih.gov/pubmed/19335713

http://www.ncbi.nlm.nih.gov/pubmed/25477716

http://www.ncbi.nlm.nih.gov/pubmed/10049982

http://www.ncbi.nlm.nih.gov/pubmed/12828188

http://www.ncbi.nlm.nih.gov/pubmed/23803881

http://www.ncbi.nlm.nih.gov/pubmed/17023705/

http://www.ncbi.nlm.nih.gov/pubmed/22826636/

http://www.ncbi.nlm.nih.gov/pubmed/20103560/

http://www.ncbi.nlm.nih.gov/pubmed/24229726

http://www.ncbi.nlm.nih.gov/pubmed/17697898

http://www.ncbi.nlm.nih.gov/pubmed/11790961

http://www.ncbi.nlm.nih.gov/pubmed/24008907/

de Munter JS, Hu FB, Spiegelman D, Franz M, van Dam RM. Whole grain, bran, and germ intake and risk of type 2 diabetes: a prospective cohort study and systematic review. PLoS Med. 2007;4:e261.

3. Beulens JW, de Bruijne LM, Stolk RP, et al. High dietary glycemic load and glycemic index increase risk of cardiovascular disease among middle-aged women: a population-based follow-up study. J Am Coll Cardiol. 2007;50:14-21.

4. Halton TL, Willett WC, Liu S, et al. Low-carbohydrate-diet score and the risk of coronary heart disease in women. N Engl J Med. 2006;355:1991-2002.

5. Anderson JW, Randles KM, Kendall CW, Jenkins DJ. Carbohydrate and fiber recommendations for individuals with diabetes: a quantitative assessment and meta-analysis of the evidence. J Am Coll Nutr. 2004;23:5-17.

6. Ebbeling CB, Leidig MM, Feldman HA, Lovesky MM, Ludwig DS. Effects of a low-glycemic load vs low-fat diet in obese young adults: a randomized trial. JAMA. 2007;297:2092-102.

7. Maki KC, Rains TM, Kaden VN, Raneri KR, Davidson MH. Effects of a reduced-glycemic-load diet on body weight, body composition, and cardiovascular disease risk markers in overweight and obese adults. Am J Clin Nutr. 2007;85:724-34.

8. Chiu CJ, Hubbard LD, Armstrong J, et al. Dietary glycemic index and carbohydrate in relation to early age-related macular degeneration. Am J Clin Nutr. 2006;83:880-6.

9. Chavarro JE, Rich-Edwards JW, Rosner BA, Willett WC. A prospective study of dietary carbohydrate quantity and quality in relation to risk of ovulatory infertility. Eur J Clin Nutr. 2009;63:78-86.

10. Higginbotham S, Zhang ZF, Lee IM, et al. Dietary glycemic load and risk of colorectal cancer in the Women's Health Study. J Natl Cancer Inst. 2004;96:229-33.

11. Liu S, Willett WC. Dietary glycemic load and atherothrombotic risk. Curr Atheroscler Rep. 2002;4:454-61.

12. Willett W, Manson J, Liu S. Glycemic index, glycemic load, and risk of type 2 diabetes. Am J Clin Nutr. 2002;76:274S-80S.

13. Livesey G, Taylor R, Livesey H, Liu S. Is there a dose-response relation of dietary glycemic load to risk of type 2 diabetes? Meta-analysis of prospective cohort studies. Am J Clin Nutr. 2013;97:584-96.

14. Mirrahimi A, de Souza RJ, Chiavaroli L, et al. Associations of glycemic index and load with coronary heart disease events: a systematic review and meta-analysis of prospective cohorts. J Am Heart Assoc. 2012;1:e000752.

15. Foster-Powell K, Holt SH, Brand-Miller JC. International table of glycemic index and glycemic load values: 2002. Am J Clin Nutr. 2002;76:5-56.

16. Buyken, AE, Goletzke, J, Joslowski, G, Felbick, A, Cheng, G, Herder, C, Brand-Miller, JC. Association between carbohydrate quality and inflammatory markers: systematic review of observational and interventional studies. The American Journal of Clinical Nutrition Am J Clin Nutr. 99(4): 2014;813-33.

17. AlEssa H, Bupathiraju S, Malik V, Wedick N, Campos H, Rosner B, Willett W, Hu FB.

Carbohydrate quality measured using multiple quality metrics is negatively associated with type 2 diabetes. Circulation. 2015; 1-31:A:20.

https://www.eatingdisorderhope.com/information/food-addiction

https://www.familyeducation.com/life/sugar/are-we-too-sweet-our-kids-addiction-sugar

https://www.coca-cola.co.uk/faq/how-much-sugar-is-in-coca-cola

https://www.today.com/health/4-rules-added-sugars-how-calculate-your-daily-limit-t34731

https://www.webmd.com/food-recipes/features/sugar-shockers-foods-surprisingly-high-in-sugar#1

https://www.diabetes.co.uk/news/2016/oct/excess-sugar-in-liver-causes-insulin-resistance,-say-researchers-91560717.html

https://www.diabetes.co.uk/insulin-resistance.html

https://articles.mercola.com/sugar-side-effects.aspx

https://integrativemedicine.arizona.edu/formalbio_rlustig.html

http://circ.ahajournals.org/content/circulationaha/120/11/1011.full.pdf

https://www.ncbi.nlm.nih.gov/pmc/articles/PMC3046985/

https://www.ncbi.nlm.nih.gov/pubmed/20413889

http://www.who.int/dietphysicalactivity/childhood/en/

http://www.who.int/dietphysicalactivity/childhood_what/en/

https://letsmove.obamawhitehouse.archives.gov/obesity

https://www.ncbi.nlm.nih.gov/pubmed/25949965

https://www.ncbi.nlm.nih.gov/pmc/articles/PMC4449512/

https://www.pediatric.theclinics.com/article/S0031-3955(11)00113-1/abstract

https://www.ncbi.nlm.nih.gov/pubmed/26194333

https://www.ncbi.nlm.nih.gov/pmc/articles/PMC3656401/

https://articles.mercola.com/sites/articles/archive/2010/04/20/sugar-dangers.aspx#_edn1

https://www.visiongain.com/Press_Release/405/Diabetes-drugs-market-will-reach-55-3bn-in-2017-with-further-growth-to-2023-predicts-Visiongain-in-new-report

https://www.perfectketo.com/fruit-on-keto/

https://www.webmd.com/food-recipes/most-important-meal#1

GENLAB Medical Diagnostics and Research Laboratory,

1 Marmara University, Engineering Faculty, Department of Chemical Engineering,

2 Marmara University, School of Physical Education and Sports – Istanbul,

3 University of Gaziantep, The School of Physical Education and Sports,

4 Firat University Medicine Faculty Biochemistry Department,

5 Muğla University The School of Physical Education and Sports, Mugla – Turkey

Correspondence to: Yrd. Doc. Dr. Kursat Karacabey, PhD

University of Gaziantep, The School of Physical Education

and Sports (Beden Egitimi ve Spor Y.O)

TR 27100, Gaziantep, TURKEY

FAX: +90 342 3600751

EMAIL: kkaracabey@gmail.com

karacabey@gantep.edu.tr

Thyroid hormones and the interrelationship of cortisol and prolactin; Influence of prolonged, exhaustive exercise

http://www.ncbi.nlm.nih.gov/pubmed/19753538

Hypothyroid myopathy. Physiopathological approach.

http://www.ncbi.nlm.nih.gov/pubmed/1339062

Thyroid hormonal responses to intensive interval versus steady state endurance exercise sessions.

http://www.ncbi.nlm.nih.gov/pubmed/?term=thyroid+hormonal+responses+to+intensive+interval+exercise

Decreased serum T3 after an exercise session is independent of glucocorticoid peak

http://www.ncbi.nlm.nih.gov/pubmed/23918684

A review of effects of hypothyroidism on vascular transport in skeletal muscle during exercise

http://www.ncbi.nlm.nih.gov/pubmed/9018403

Human mitochondrial transcription factor (A) reduction and mitochondrial dysfunction in

hashimoto's hypothyroid myopathy

http://www.ncbi.nlm.nih.gov/pubmed/?term=human+mitochondrial+transcription+a+reduction+and+mitochondrial+dysfunction++in+Hashimoto%27s

Spence JD, Jenkins DJ, Davignon J. 2010. "Dietary cholesterol and egg yolks: not for patients at risk of vascular disease." Canadian Journal of Cardiology, November 26.

2. U.S. Food and Drug Administration. 2009. FDA Improves Egg Safety.

3. Anderson KE. 2011. "Comparison of fatty acid, cholesterol, and vitamin A and E composition in eggs from hens housed in conventional cage and range production facilities." Poultry Science, July.

4. Djoussé L, Gaziano JM. 2008. "Egg consumption in relation to cardiovascular disease and mortality: the Physicians' Health Study." American Journal of Clinical Nutrition, April.

http://www.mayoclinic.com/health/legumes/NU00260

http://jcem.endojournals.org/content/88/10/4857.abstract

http://www.krispin.com/lectin.html

http://www.marksdailyapple.com/lectins/

http://en.wikipedia.org/wiki/Legume

https://www.ncbi.nlm.nih.gov/pmc/articles/PMC2121650/

https://www.ncbi.nlm.nih.gov/pmc/articles/PMC3391950/

https://www.ncbi.nlm.nih.gov/pmc/articles/PMC3773450/

https://www.ncbi.nlm.nih.gov/pmc/articles/PMC4049200/

https://www.ncbi.nlm.nih.gov/pmc/articles/PMC4390184/

https://www.ncbi.nlm.nih.gov/pmc/articles/PMC4409470/

https://www.ncbi.nlm.nih.gov/pmc/articles/PMC4808863/

https://www.ncbi.nlm.nih.gov/pubmed/23026007

https://www.ncbi.nlm.nih.gov/pubmed/3899519

https://www.registerednursing.org/nclex/fluid-electrolyte-imbalances/

https://www.medicalnewstoday.com/articles/153188.php

articles.mercola.com/.../organic-psyllium-husk.aspx

healthline.com/.../magnesium-for-citrate-constipation

https://www.healthline.com/health/electrolyte-disorders#causes

http://chemocare.com/chemotherapy/side-effects/electrolyte-imbalance.aspx

https://www.emedicinehealth.com/electrolytes/article_em.htm

https://www.livestrong.com/article/216779-how-do-i-correct-an-electrolyte-imbalance/

https://www.organicfacts.net/electrolyte-imbalance.html

http://cancer.unm.edu/cancer/cancer-info/cancer-treatment/side-effects-of-cancer-treatment/less-common-side-effects/blood-test-abnormalities/electrolyte-imbalance/

https://myhealth.alberta.ca/Health/aftercareinformation/pages/conditions.aspx?hwid=bz1133http://www.foodnetwork.com/healthyeats/2012/07/staying-hydrated-electrolytes-101

https://www.rodalewellness.com/food/food-for-fitness-electrolytes/slide/3

http://agris.fao.org/agris-search/search.do?recordID=US201303016467

https://draxe.com/pink-himalayan-salt/

https://www.medicalnewstoday.com/articles/153188.php

articles.mercola.com/.../organic-psyllium-husk.aspx

healthline.com/.../magnesium-for-citrate-constipation

https://www.healthline.com/health/electrolyte-disorders#causes

http://chemocare.com/chemotherapy/side-effects/electrolyte-imbalance.aspx

https://www.emedicinehealth.com/electrolytes/article_em.htm

https://www.livestrong.com/article/216779-how-do-i-correct-an-electrolyte-imbalance/

https://www.organicfacts.net/electrolyte-imbalance.html

http://cancer.unm.edu/cancer/cancer-info/cancer-treatment/side-effects-of-cancer-treatment/less-common-side-effects/blood-test-abnormalities/electrolyte-imbalance/

https://myhealth.alberta.ca/Health/aftercareinformation/pages/conditions.aspx?hwid=bz1133

http://www.foodnetwork.com/healthyeats/2012/07/staying-hydrated-electrolytes-101

https://www.rodalewellness.com/food/food-for-fitness-electrolytes/slide/3

http://agris.fao.org/agris-search/search.do?recordID=US201303016467

https://draxe.com/pink-himalayan-salt/

https://www.registerednursing.org/nclex/fluid-electrolyte-imbalances/

http://www.accessdata.fda.gov/scripts/Plantox/Detail.CFM?ID=6537

Barceloux DG 2009. Potatoes, tomatoes, and solanine toxicity. Dis Mon 55(6):391-402.

Friedman M. Tomato glycoalkaloids: role in the plant and in the diet. J Agric Food Chem2002; 50:5751-5780. UDSA, Albany California.

Hansen AA. Two fatal cases of potato poisoning. Science 1925; 61(1578): 340-341.

Jones PG and Fenwick GR 1981. The glycoalkaloid content of some edible solanaceous fruits and potato products. Journal of the Science of Food and Agriculture 32(4):419-421.

Korpan YI et al. Potato glycoalkaloids: true safety or false sense of security? Trends in Biotechnology 2004; 22(3): 147-151.


McMillan M and Thompson JC. An outbreak of suspected solanine poisoning in schoolboys: examinations of criteria of solanine poisoning. Q J Med 1979; 48(190): 227-243.

Mensinga TT et al. Potato glycoalkaloids and adverse effects in humans: an ascending dose study. Regulatory Toxicology and Pharmacology 2005;41: 66-72. University of Utrecht, The Netherlands.

Milner SE et al. Bioactivities of glycoalkaloids and their aglycones from Solanum species. J Agric Food Chem 2011; 59: 3454-3484. University College, Cork Ireland.

Patel B et al. Potato glycoalkaloids adversely affect intestinal permeability and aggravate inflammatory bowel disease. Inflammatory Bowel Diseases 2002; 8 (5): 340-346.

Sanchez-Mata MC et al. r-Solasonine and r-Solamargine Contents of Gboma (Solanum macrocarpon L.) and Scarlet (Solanum aethiopicum L.) Eggplants J Agric Food Chem 2010; 58: 5502-5508.

Siegmund B et al. Determination of the nicotine content of various edible nightshades (Solanaceae) and their products and estimation of the associated dietary nicotine intake. J Agric Food Chem 1999;47: 3113-3120.

https://www.livestrong.com/article/305368-list-of-foods-that-contain-lectin/

https://www.ncbi.nlm.nih.gov/books/NBK22545/

https://www.ncbi.nlm.nih.gov/pubmed/1824332

https://www.selfhacked.com/blog/elimination-diet-safest-foods-people-sensitive-everything/

http://articles.mercola.com/sites/articles/archive/2014/02/24/dry-skin-brushing.aspx

https://health.clevelandclinic.org/2015/01/the-truth-about-dry-brushing-and-what-it-does-for-you/

http://www.mamamia.com.au/slimming-body-wraps-danger/

http://goop.com/how-to-dry-brush-and-why-its-so-potent/

http://blackdoctor.org/483081/the-dangers-of-wrapping-plastic-wrap-around-your-belly/2/

http://www.accessdata.fda.gov/scripts/Plantox/Detail.CFM?ID=6537

Barceloux DG 2009. Potatoes, tomatoes, and solanine toxicity. Dis Mon 55(6):391-402.

Friedman M. Tomato glycoalkaloids: role in the plant and in the diet. J Agric Food Chem2002; 50:5751-5780. UDSA, Albany California.

Hansen AA. Two fatal cases of potato poisoning. Science 1925; 61(1578): 340-341.

Jones PG and Fenwick GR 1981. The glycoalkaloid content of some edible solanaceous fruits and potato products. Journal of the Science of Food and Agriculture 32(4):419-421.

Korpan YI et al. Potato glycoalkaloids: true safety or false sense of security? Trends in Biotechnology 2004; 22(3): 147-151.

McMillan M and Thompson JC. An outbreak of suspected solanine poisoning in schoolboys: examinations of criteria of solanine poisoning. Q J Med 1979; 48(190): 227-243.

Mensinga TT et al. Potato glycoalkaloids and adverse effects in humans: an ascending dose study. Regulatory Toxicology and Pharmacology 2005;41: 66-72. University of Utrecht, The Netherlands.

Milner SE et al. Bioactivities of glycoalkaloids and their aglycones from Solanum species. J Agric Food Chem 2011; 59: 3454-3484. University College, Cork Ireland.

Patel B et al. Potato glycoalkaloids adversely affect intestinal permeability and aggravate inflammatory bowel disease. Inflammatory Bowel Diseases 2002; 8 (5): 340-346.

Sanchez-Mata MC et al. r-Solasonine and r-Solamargine Contents of Gboma (Solanum macrocarpon L.) and Scarlet (Solanum aethiopicum L.) Eggplants J Agric Food Chem 2010; 58: 5502-5508.

Siegmund B et al.  Determination of the nicotine content of various edible nightshades (Solanaceae) and their products and estimation of the associated dietary nicotine intake.  J Agric Food Chem 1999;47: 3113–3120.

https://www.livestrong.com/article/305368-list-of-foods-that-contain-lectin/

Made in the USA
Columbia, SC
01 September 2022